BAG

BAG

THE ULTIMATE FASHION
ACCESSORY

Sue Huey   Susie Draffan

Laurence King Publishing

Published in 2009.
This edition published in 2013 by
Laurence King Publishing Ltd
361–373 City Road
London EC1V 1LR
United Kingdom
Tel: +44 20 7841 6900
Fax: +44 20 7841 6910
email: enquiries@laurenceking.com
www.laurenceking.com

A catalogue record for this book is available from
the British Library.

ISBN: 978 1 78067 019 5

Design: byBOTH

Project editor: Gaynor Sermon
Project assistance: Claire Murphy and Alison Bishop

Commissioned photography:
John-Paul Pietrus www.johnpaulpietrus.com
Retouching and digital artwork:
Nick Nedeljkovic www.happyfinish.com

Printed in China

LOVE
BAGS

It is a widely acknowledged Fashion Fact that there are two items in a woman's wardrobe that she should invest in, pieces that are classic yet instantly update an outfit, and are financially justifiable as they will be kept forever and worn again and again: one is a coat, and the other is a handbag.

It is impossible to overstate the significance of a handbag to a woman. More than just a repository for our day-to-day essentials, a bag becomes an extension of ourselves – it holds our lives, our everyday worlds. Someone who realized the importance of this was Gabrielle Chanel, who created a hidden pocket in the interior of her iconic 2.55 bag, in which to keep 'a woman's secrets'.

Bags become our favoured possessions, our trusted allies – we take them everywhere with us and often have one for every occasion. Grace Kelly famously used hers to hide a pregnant stomach, prompting Hermès to rename the bag in her honour; Jessica Simpson infamously asked if it was weird to take her Louis Vuitton bag camping; Kate Moss reportedly owns a jaw-dropping 100 CHANEL bags.

A woman's choice of handbag speaks volumes about her: it projects an image, revealing who she is and who she would like to be. A bag can bring out our obsessive natures, betraying a compulsion to possess a little piece of luxury, and it has the power to inspire jealousy and desire. Anyone who's suffered from 'handbag envy' knows it can produce a yearning equal to that of any star-crossed lovers! Women judge each other by their bags, and the bag that you carry can say more about who you are than any other item in your wardrobe.

This book is about the love of bags. It is not about the history of the bag, or the luxury industry of which bags and accessories are a major part, or even about IT bags, which are a modern phenomenon. Rather, it celebrates the very best of beautiful, covetable, lust-worthy design. The designers featured in these pages include classic, long-standing brands that have stood the test of time, such as Hermès and CHANEL; brands that have been established in the last 20 years, including Dolce&Gabbana and Jamin Puech, who excel at bag design and have made a name for themselves in the world of luxury accessories by designing the classics of the future; new labels who are making an impact on bag design and carving out their own niche in the market, such as Isaac Reina and Phillip Lim. What all of these designers and brands have in common is a commitment to craftsmanship and quality materials, and to creating beautiful bags that women quite simply fall in love with.

'IT BAGS GENERALLY HAVE VERY LITTLE BRANDING AND ARE OFTEN UNDERSTATED, IT WAS ALL ABOUT DESIGN. THE DESIGN IS WHAT MAKES A BAG SPECIAL, EVERYONE IN THE KNOW KNOWS HOW MUCH THE PIECE COST SO YOU STILL HAVE THE STATUS, IT'S LIKE BEING PART OF A COOL GANG.'

The handbag has come a long way since its humble beginnings as a pouch to carry coins. By the 12th century it had moved a step closer to its current incarnation, as the first 'designer' pouch was created in leather in Italy, and by the time of the Belle Epoque at the end of the 19th century the pouch had transformed itself into something that we would recognize today.

Even though it has changed its appearance numerous times over the centuries, the handbag has never gone out of style. Even Diana Vreeland, the legendary Editor-in-Chief of American *Vogue*, announcing in the 1950s that

'we are going to eliminate all handbags'

couldn't persuade women to give up this treasured possession, and half a century later we are ever more in their thrall, raising handbags to the level of icons, creating a phenomenon out of the 'bag of the moment'.

Stuart Vevers, Creative Director of Loewe, believes that

'The bag became a status symbol for those in the know. It generally wasn't about branding, or even status, quite the opposite: IT bags generally have very little branding and are often understated, it was all about design. The design is what makes a bag special, everyone in the know knows how much the piece cost so you still have the status, it's like being part of a cool gang.'

In recent years it has been proven time and again that a label's profile can be raised enormously through celebrity endorsements. Capture the right bag on the right girl at the right time and you can create a feverish frenzy that ensures you have a 'hit' bag on your hands. What makes an 'IT bag', however, cannot be clearly defined: there are many different types of IT bag, from the obvious – featuring excessive hardware and brand logos that are instantly recognizable and scream status – to the low key but no less luxurious bags that focus on quality and craftsmanship. But fashion moves fast and the quest for the new means that IT bags are often tied to one season and date quickly.

The internet is flooded with websites and blogs celebrating the latest designer bags, salivating over everything from the suppleness of the leather and the quality of the top stitching to the shininess of the hardware. There are social networking sites for handbag lovers, online communities where like-minded bag aficionados share their enthusiasms, and on websites such as ebay thousands of bidders play a game of cat and mouse in online auctions of designer handbags and vintage purses. Bags

'I LOVE ALL OF MY BAGS AND THAT'S BECAUSE I PURCHASED THEM WITH EMOTION. I FEEL THAT, ESSENTIALLY, THAT IS WHAT A WOMAN WANTS TO FEEL, A SPECIAL EMOTION FOR THE INVESTMENT SHE MAKES. THIS WAY SHE WILL TREASURE HER BAGS FOREVER.'

now have cult followings and the demand for them can make even the sanest person go crazy: when Anya Hindmarch launched her 'I'm Not a Plastic Bag' eco-friendly tote in Taiwan, for example, riot police were called in to manage the crowds.

While demand for the next must-have bag – from the Chloé Paddington to the Marc Jacobs Stam – has persisted from the beginning of the decade, there now seems to be a move towards quieter, more understated luxury.

'I think we are more willing to invest in luxury, choosing to spend on investment pieces with longevity and are becoming less interested in throwaway fashion,'

says Anya Hindmarch.

'I would rather own something luxurious and perhaps "seasonless" that I feel will be cherished for a lifetime than many pieces I will soon tire of.'

The future of the IT bag is uncertain. Some are predicting that the phenomena has run its course, while others believe there is still room for it in the market. In the end, what makes a bag a success is a mixture of timing, luck and, ultimately, a woman's emotional connection with it.

'I think that longevity is always key,'

says Tia Cibani of Ports 1961.

'I love all of my bags and that's because I purchased them with emotion. I feel that, essentially, that is what a woman wants to feel, a special emotion for the investment she makes. This way she will treasure her bags forever.'

These days bags come in myriad shapes and sizes, from teeny lipstick purses to cavernous slouchy sack-bags, and are made from all manner of materials, from Rocio's intricately carved wooden clutches, inlaid with precious stones, to Zagliani's vibrantly coloured totes fashioned from exotic crocodile- and snakeskins made sensationally supple with the injection of cosmetic 'fillers'. Whatever your taste, you can be assured there exists the perfect bag for you: you may even discover yours within the pages of this book, where modern classics like Marc Jacobs' Stam nestle alongside favourites such as the Hermès Birkin and the CHANEL 2.55; where styles range from Jas M.B's fiercely functional messenger bags to Port 1961's sculpted works of art, and from stunningly simple Halston Sacs to wittily embellished Moschino arm candy. Bag yourself a little piece of handbag heaven.

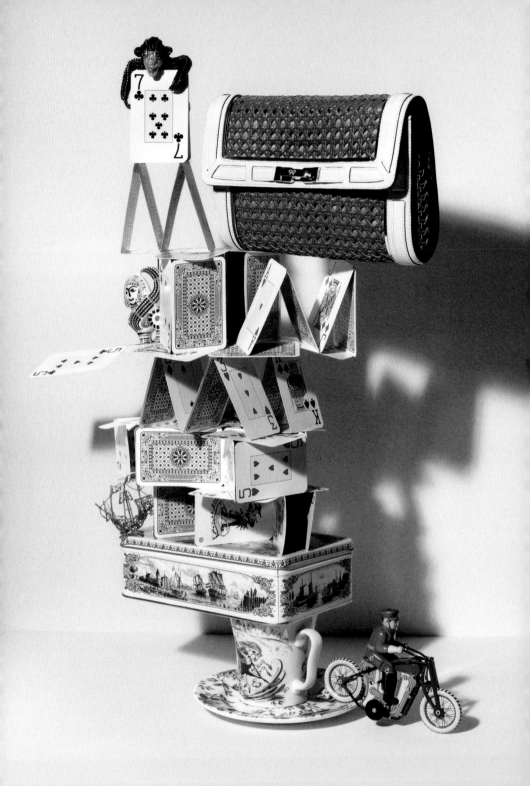

ANYA HINDMARCH

A globally recognized British brand that retains its
niche appeal, Anya Hindmarch has grown from a small
London boutique to 46 stores worldwide. From her
groundbreaking 'I'm Not a Plastic Bag' campaign to
her luxurious Bespoke Ebury bags, Hindmarch has
made her mark at both ends of the market.

OPPOSITE Capsule clutch in tan wicker-chair leather,
S/S 09.

Founded in 1991
www.anyahindmarch.com

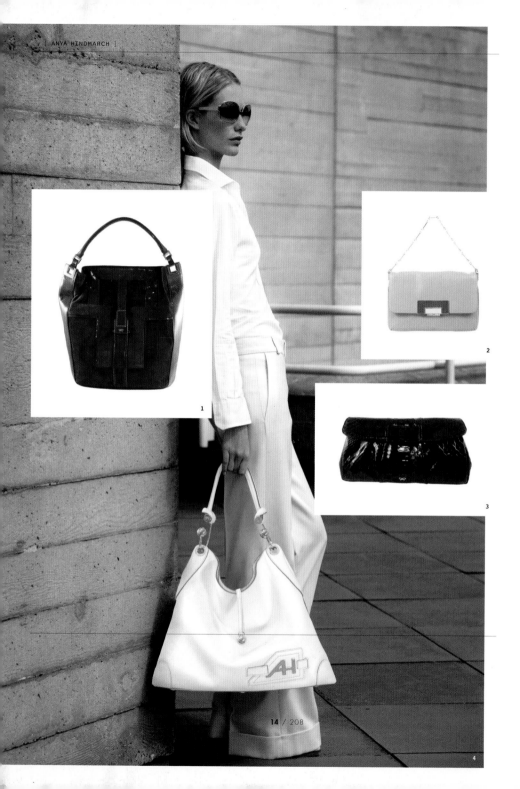

1

2

3

4

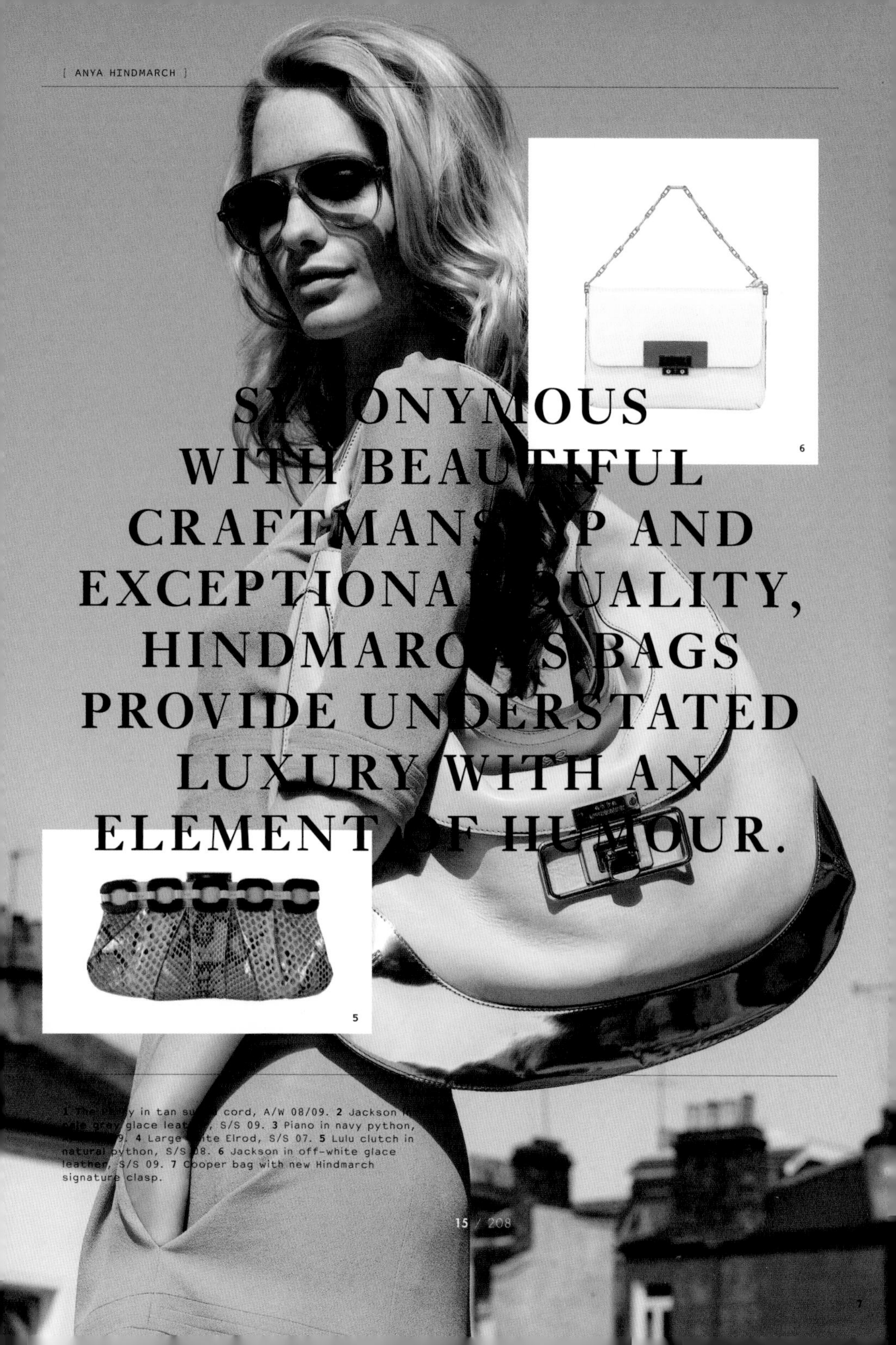

SYNONYMOUS
WITH BEAUTIFUL
CRAFTMANSHIP AND
EXCEPTIONAL QUALITY,
HINDMARCH'S BAGS
PROVIDE UNDERSTATED
LUXURY WITH AN
ELEMENT OF HUMOUR.

1 The Jimmy in tan suede cord, A/W 08/09. 2 Jackson in pale grey glace leather, S/S 09. 3 Piano in navy python, S/S 09. 4 Large white Elrod, S/S 07. 5 Lulu clutch in natural python, S/S 08. 6 Jackson in off-white glace leather, S/S 09. 7 Cooper bag with new Hindmarch signature clasp.

7

Designing since she was four years old, one of Anya Hindmarch's greatest strengths is that, as a modern working women, she is perfectly in-tune with her market and knows exactly what women want – whether that is a beautifully crafted leather bag, a bespoke piece with a secret message embossed in the interior or a socially responsible canvas tote.

Creating a sensation in 2007 when she launched her limited edition 'I'm Not a Plastic Bag' tote in collaboration with the global social change movement We Are What We Do, Hindmarch used her status as a well-known designer for positive change. 'I'm Not a Plastic Bag' promoted the use of reusable canvas shoppers as an alternative to environmentally unfriendly plastic bags. Retailing at £5 (US $7.50), they sold out within hours and quickly became one of the most covetable and talked-about bags of the past decade.

Hindmarch has twice been honoured with the British Fashion Awards Designer Brand of the Year award, and also designs shoes, luggage, and a small ready-to-wear collection.

How did you initially get into bag design?

'I started the business after living in Florence when I was nineteen. I noticed that the drawstring, leather duffel bag was a strong trend amongst Florentine women and when I returned to England, I approached *Harper's & Queen* about a special commission. I designed a bag for a special offer for the magazine; 500 were sold and the Anya Hindmarch brand was born. I come from a family of entrepreneurs so it was natural for me to want to start my own business. Both my brother and sister have their own businesses. When I started I also saw a gap in the market for bags that were a bit more creative and special.'

Do you have a certain process when working on the collection?

'I design with myself in mind. Women play many different roles now: we work, travel, have families and we still like to enjoy ourselves. I think I have the experience to make a bag that is right in all these roles!'

Can you describe your techniques?

'I think fabric, cut and design combine to make a handbag great, but attention to detail makes a handbag special. I am obsessed with bespoke and love surprise touches, both personal and practical — lipstick pouches and detachable key fobs — these are what make a bag unique and something to treasure.'

What is your signature design style?

'I am interested in great craftsmanship, beautiful materials, proportion, attention to detail and creating something beyond the expected. I think I design bags that are luxurious and serve their purpose with a touch of humour. Accessories truly punctuate how you project yourself and can be more important than clothing. They are the defining part of an outfit, I think. I love the way that a handbag can change the way that a woman feels.'

What inspires you?

'I am inspired by all sorts of things, memories of my mother's outfits in the 1970s, Slim Aaron's pictures of beautiful socialites. I often find that I am inspired by architecture. I am obsessed by modern architecture and the period in the late 1950s is a particular source of fascination for me.'

What materials/fabrications do you use?

'I love beautiful rich materials like calfskin, python, cashmere, satin. I also use crocodile, eel and rabbit occasionally.'

What are your plans and ambitions for the future?

'Many things I am sure I have not yet even thought of.'

How do you feel about the industry at the moment and how do you think it is going to develop in the future?

'I think the way we think about accessories is changing. I think we are more willing to invest in luxury, choosing to spend on investment pieces with longevity, and are becoming less interested in throwaway fashion. I would rather own something luxurious and perhaps "seasonless" that I feel will be cherished for a lifetime than many pieces I will soon tire of.'

OPPOSITE Bespoke Ebury in blue calf leather.

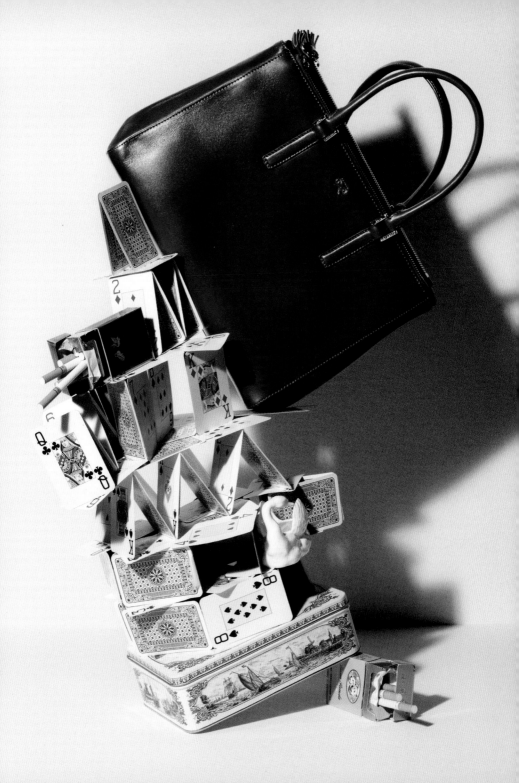

An independent American brand with a
devoted global fan base, Botkier combines
luxury with a stylish practicality. This
winning formula has earned the brand
success Stateside and beyond.

BOTKIER

OPPOSITE Holiday resort collection, 2008.

Founded in 2003
www.botkier.com

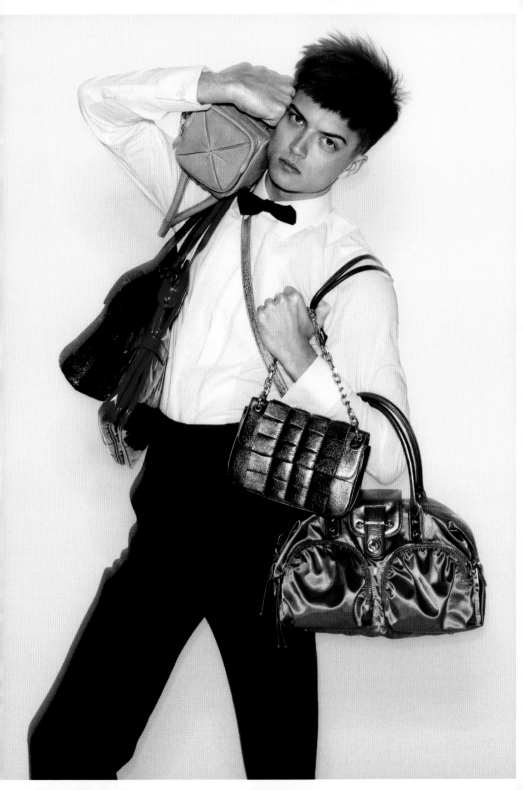

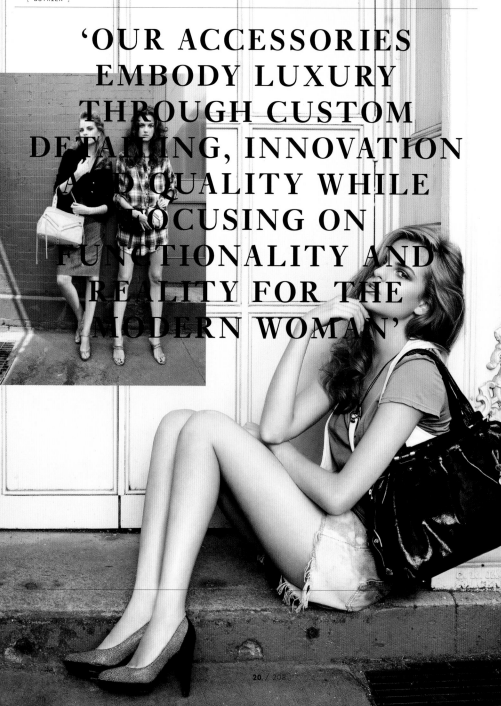

'OUR ACCESSORIES EMBODY LUXURY THROUGH CUSTOM DETAILING, INNOVATION AND QUALITY WHILE FOCUSING ON FUNCTIONALITY AND REALITY FOR THE MODERN WOMAN'

Native New Yorker Monica Botkier has always had a keen eye for fashion – and in particular accessories. Her personal quest to design the perfect handbag was so well received by industry friends and fashion editors that she decided to launch her own fashion label, Botkier, in 2003. Having previously worked as a photographer for magazines such as *Surface* and *Mademoiselle*, Monica continues to pursue photography by shooting Botkier advertising campaigns each season, thus marrying her love of fashion with her passion for photography.

Describing her style as 'approachable', Botkier believes the label's overnight success has in part been a result of its unique market position. By creating a fashion niche where there was once a void, and setting price points just below those of high-end designer labels, Botkier is able to offer affordable luxury.

'Our accessories embody luxury through custom detailing, innovation and quality while focusing on functionality and reality for the modern woman', Monica Botkier explains.

Botkier's style very much reflects its origins, and successfully marries a downtown Manhattan look with a functional utilitarian edge. This style is defined perfectly by signature bag styles such as the Trigger, the Bianca and the Sasha. While hugely practical, the Botkier bag is always stylish, popular as much for its attention to detail as for its subtle branding. Slouchy silhouettes are combined with intricate construction and handcrafted leather detailing such as gathers, pleats and ruching, while colours and supple leathers are offered in both classic and more daring combinations.

This look has struck a chord with some of the world's most recognized celebrities. Angelina Jolie, Jessica Alba, Lindsay Lohan, Heidi Klum, Joy Bryant and Kate Bosworth are among Botkier's most acclaimed admirers. A celebrity following of this scale is often the creation of a bestselling bag, but while Monica Botkier and her bags enjoy the media spotlight she remains pragmatic, saying

'the IT bag will come and go and come back again. Women like to have a choice and be individual, but the allure of that bag that hits the mark for so many is always out there.'

Inspired by the local surroundings of her Manhattan lifestyle, Botkier has no problem generating new design ideas.

'Life is always inspiring if you just take the time to look around',

she believes, citing travel, antique jewellery, leather and photography as her main sources of inspiration.

Botkier's approach to design follows no particular order from season to season,

'the process is different for every collection',

she claims. Sketching, collecting and listening to music all contribute to the design process, allowing her to piece her thoughts and ideas together to create narratives and identities for each of her forty-something styles. By choosing to use custom-made leathers and hardware specifically created for the brand, Botkier also seeks perfection in her work, saying

'There is something exciting about hardware and leather; this synergy creates a direct and easy way to express oneself, you can take risks wearing a Botkier accessory and push the envelope daily.'

Challenging her customers is part of the wider Botkier philosophy of creating the ideal bag while at the same time tackling new markets:

'The market is quite saturated, which is a good thing. Women's needs won't change but a more competitive retail environment will bring out the best in solid designers and weed out the brands we don't need.'

Having already launched a shoe- and a leather goods range, Botkier has big plans for the future, which include turning the Botkier accessory experience into a retail reality.

'I love leather and all things accessory, so we will continue to build upon our success and grow by making our philosophy global.'

MAIN PICTURE Violet large satchel, S/S 09. **INSET** Trigger bags, S/S 09.

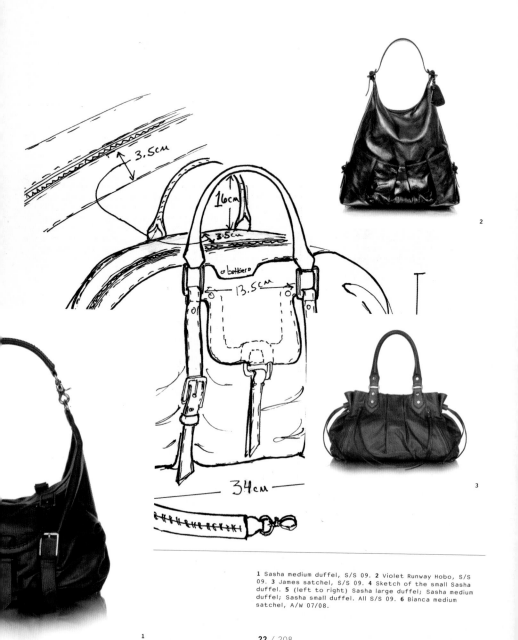

1 Sasha medium duffel, S/S 09. 2 Violet Runway Hobo, S/S
09. 3 James satchel, S/S 09. 4 Sketch of the small Sasha
duffel. 5 (left to right) Sasha large duffel; Sasha medium
duffel; Sasha small duffel. All S/S 09. 6 Bianca medium
satchel, A/W 07/08.

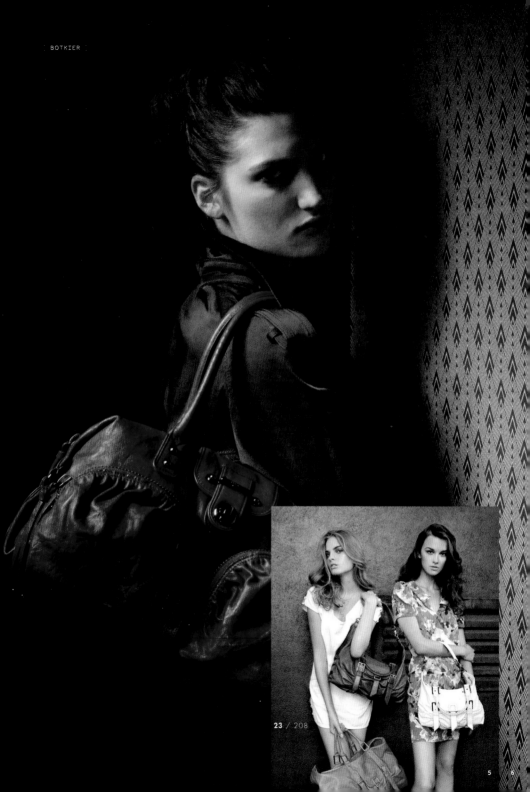

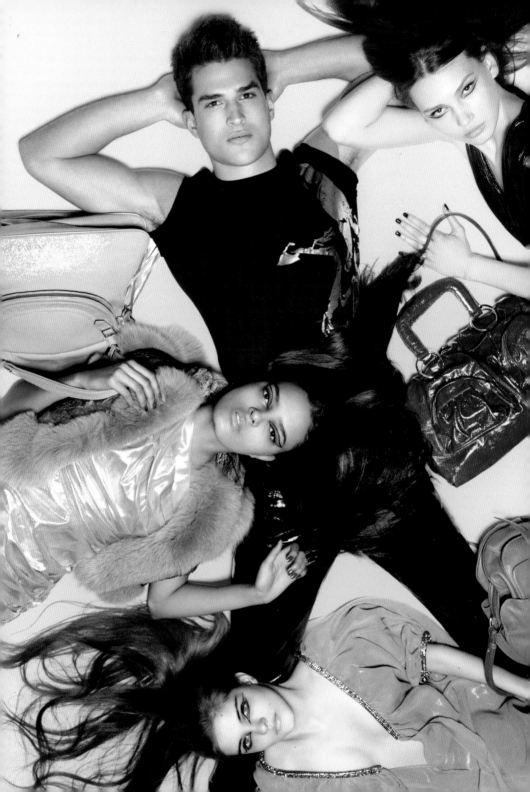

BULGA

Working with soft leather shapes and silhouettes, Bulga is known for its elegant, stylish and weightless handbags and has become recognized as a pioneer of affordable designer style.

CLOCKWISE FROM TOP LEFT 4116 crinkled patent bag, nude, S/S 08; 4230 crinkled patent purple Misa bag, A/W 08/09; 4129 Helmut bag in taupe, A/W 08/09.

Founded in 2003
www.bulgausa.com

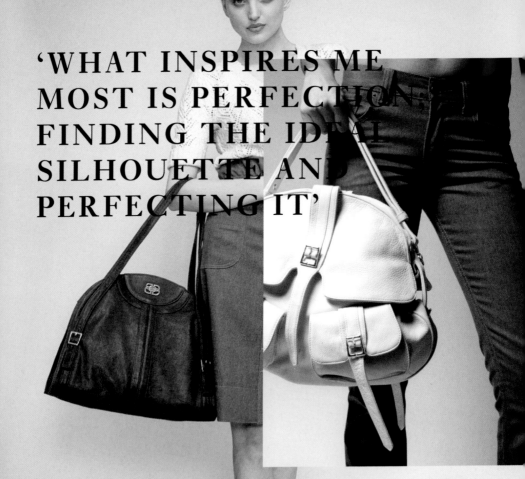

'WHAT INSPIRES ME
MOST IS PERFECTION.
FINDING THE IDEAL
SILHOUETTE AND
PERFECTING IT'

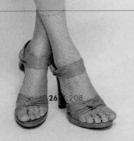

Natalia Konovalova, designer and Creative Director of New York-based label Bulga, founded the company after graduating from the Fashion Institute of Technology, and has built a reputation for modern, functional and classic designs.

The word 'bulga' derives from ancient French and Latin, and translates as a small leather- or money bag. Drawing inspiration from both her European upbringing and fast-paced New York City lifestyle, Konovalova's philosophy is to create luxury products that combine quality and originality. With its soft leather shapes and silhouettes, Bulga is known for its elegant, stylish and weightless handbags that are smart and functional with a cool, bohemian edge.

The label's colourful designs feature layering techniques and gold-plated hardware details which add a twist to otherwise classic styles. Konovalova works with fine Italian leather and custom hardware, and each bag is proudly handcrafted in New York.

Konovalova's other inspiration comes from magazines, travel, collaborating with her team and keeping a sharp eye on the catwalks as well as drawing influence from the streets.

'It is almost like a sixth sense',
explains Konovalova,
'of what is going to be in fashion and then reinterpreting it into my own vision of colours, silhouettes and designs.'

The design process involves observation and sketching, taking an initial idea and developing it into the perfect representation of the label's ideals.

'The creative process does not stop until the very end. Based on the season and the theme we order leather from Italy — that takes a couple of months — and by the time it arrives we have our first proto bags, after that we finish new bags in the key looks.'

Konovalova's favourite part of the design process is the interaction with the clients, talking to them about the collection at shows, getting their feedback and seeing their reactions first hand.

The designer's background in fashion informs Bulga's designs, through the use of tailoring and draping.

'Draped is not really a term used for handbags but I use this technique a lot. I think this way each style is more personalized. Bags can say so much about a woman — just like shoes or perfume.'

Bulga's signature bag is the studded 2934 Bag, which was inspired by a vintage dress and butterfly-like cut-outs, and became an instant hit. The designer explains:

'When it came out there was nothing like it on the market. Hobos with drawstrings were forgotten and left alone in the 1970s, we revived this look and made it cool again.'

The Bulga label has attracted a strong celebrity following, and Konovalova has ambitions to build her brand beyond bags into a full Bulga lifestyle range. Meanwhile, she sees a shift away from the current trend for IT bags to bags that offer more classic luxury, quality and functionality – much like Bulga itself.

'Everything goes in cycles and it could stay in the luxury cycle for years',
she explains.
'Then there will be those designers who come along and change it again, possibly for aesthetic reasons, or maybe because of social changes. Who knows, the next cycle could involve designers going green with their accessory designs.'

MAIN PICTURE Gabanna bag, A/W 08/09. INSET 4129 bag, A/W 08/09. OVER THE PAGE 1 4129 London, A/W 08/09. 2 Development sketch, S/S 06. 3&6 Marque bags, A/W 08/09. 4 Femour bag, A/W 09/10. 5 Gabanna Hobo, A/W 08/09.

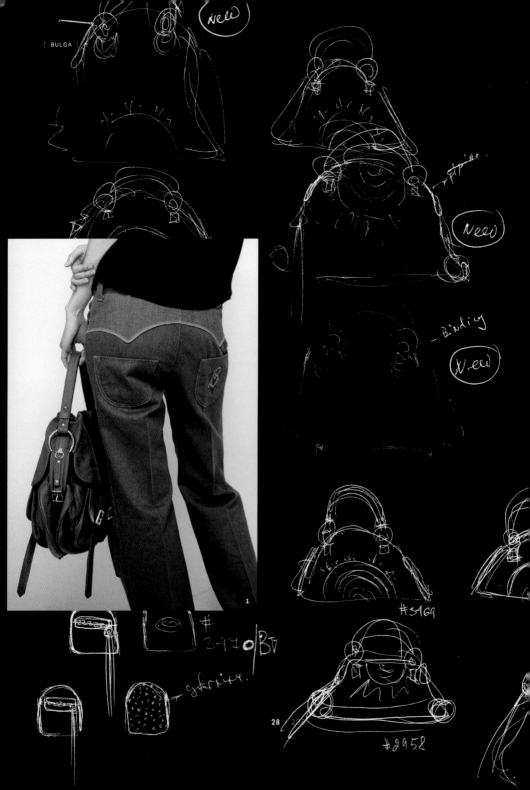

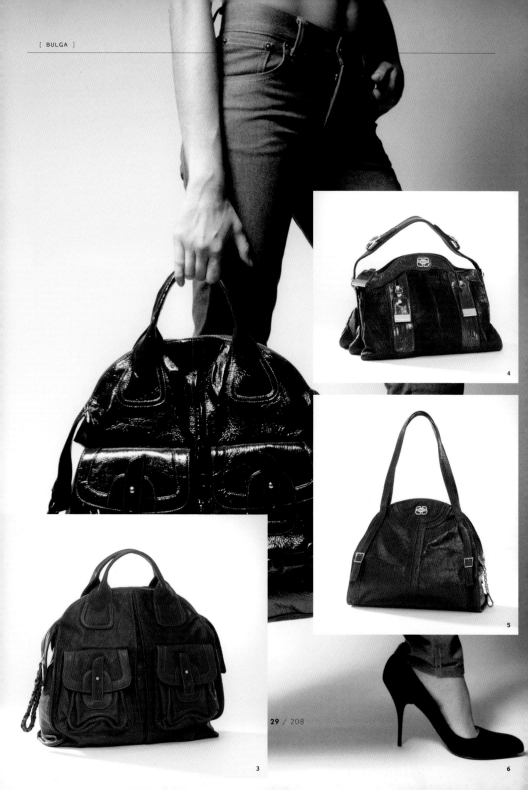

4

5

3

6

BURBERRY

Burberry is the quintessential British luxury brand. For over 150 years it has been associated with English sophistication, classic tailoring, quality and a very British sense of style.

OPPOSITE Spike clutch bag.

Founded in 1856
www.burberry.com

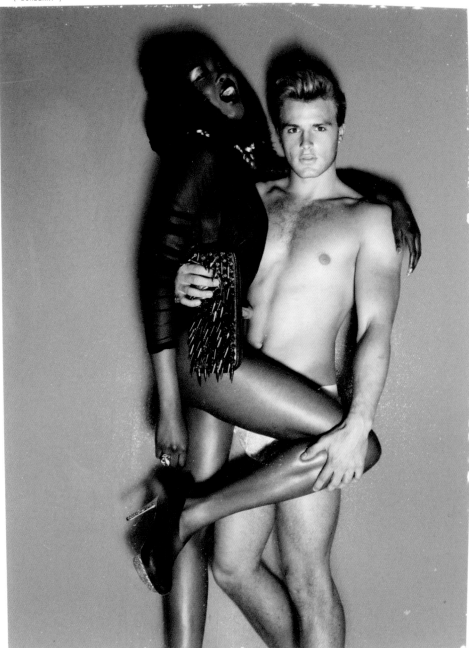

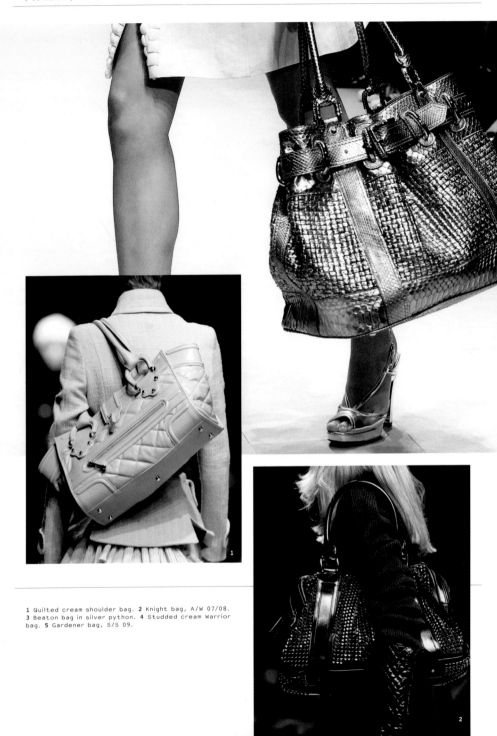

1 Quilted cream shoulder bag. 2 Knight bag, A/W 07/08.
3 Beaton bag in silver python. 4 Studded cream Warrior
bag. 5 Gardener bag, S/S 09.

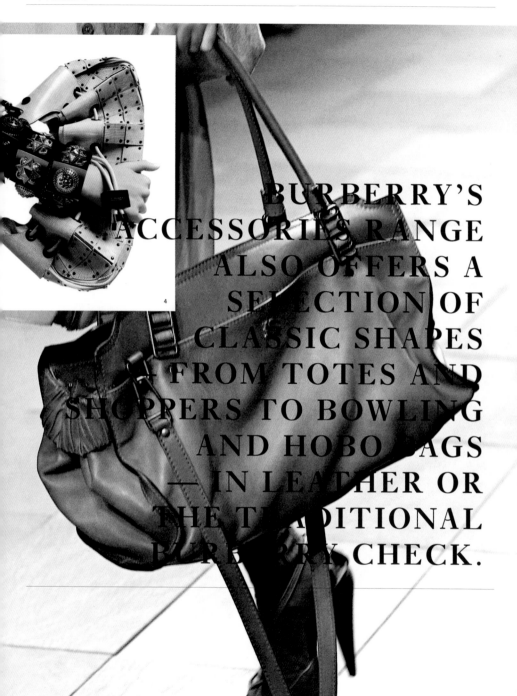

4

BURBERRY'S ACCESSORIES RANGE ALSO OFFERS A SELECTION OF CLASSIC SHAPES — FROM TOTES AND SHOPPERS TO BOWLING AND HOBO BAGS — IN LEATHER OR THE TRADITIONAL BURBERRY CHECK.

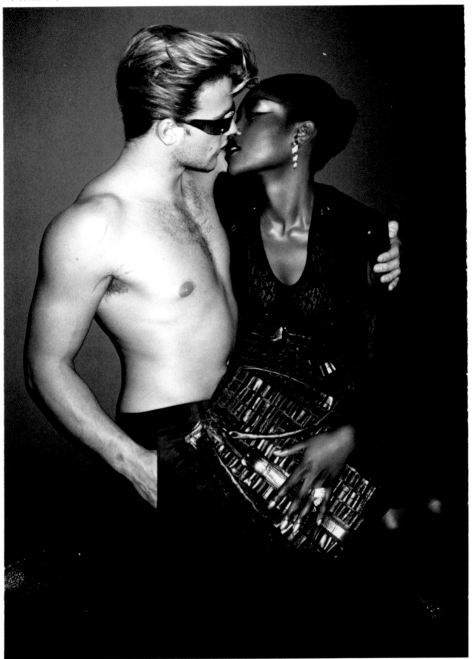

Burberry is a global brand for the 21st century, creating modern designs that play on the label's unique heritage and are desired the world over. Taking inspiration from historical British icons, British artists and the colours and landscapes of the British countryside, Burberry is a luxury brand that is British through and through.

Burberry was founded in 1856 by Thomas Burberry, a twenty-one-year-old draper's apprentice in Basingstoke, England, who had ambitions beyond those of a gentlemans' outfitters. Calling himself a 'dress reformer', Burberry innovated the field of material construction when he developed the Gabardine fabric in 1880. This dedication to innovation in both style and function would later become the company's signature.

Famous for its iconic check pattern, Burberry has in recent years undergone a renaissance at the hands of Creative Director Christopher Bailey, who has turned this classic heritage brand into a billion-pound global business and one of the most desirable fashion labels in the world. The beautiful designs with discreet detailing speak of an easy, dishevelled elegance and are beloved by city- and country folk alike, as well as new generations of young hipsters.

Burberry accessories also benefit from greater focus under Bailey's direction. Utilizing Burberry's iconic trademark check, quilting and the D-ring buckle (taken from the classic Burberry trenchcoat's belt detail), the accessories collection takes its cue from each runway collection, using details such as studded plates and Celtic-inspired metal studs.

The Lowry bag – a key piece from the Autumn/Winter 08/09 collection – is inspired by the mood, spirit and colour palette of British painter LS Lowry. Sumptuous, structured and beautifully crafted, the Lowry bag was created in a range of fabrics, including pleated alligator, ruched ribbon iguana, suede with metal stitches and sprayed textured leather. Containing fitted pockets for holding mobile phones, MP3 players and PDAs, it follows Burberry's tradition for function as well as form. The colour palette of the Lowry bag collection echoes the muted but rich tones of the Autumn/Winter 08/09 ready-to-wear pieces, from dark ochre to racing green and rich bordeaux.

Clutches offer glamour for evening and are heavily embellished, featuring faceted glass, studded plates, feathers or pleated details that echo the pleating on the Lowry bag.

For Spring/Summer 09 the clothing collection took inspiration from gardening girls and romance, featuring a gentle landscape-inspired colour palette and crumpled classics. For the bags this translated into easy-to-wear totes in textured leather with contrasting leather straps or rough-edged woven straw, trimmed in crocodile skin with buckle detailing, which epitomized 'rough luxe'. All-over crocodile and metallic versions in matt bronze and silver also featured, alongside elegant clutches.

Crocodile skin featured strongly in the Autumn/Winter 09/10 collection. Inspired by British icons, from Elizabeth, the Countess of Devon, to Virginia Woolf, Christopher Bailey mixed country and city references to create bags of understated luxury. Handheld totes are made from crocodile skin with chain drawstrings and overstitched detailing on the handles. Other fabrications include soft suede with stitched patterning, and oversized check with crocodile leather trims, straps and handles.

Burberry's accessories range features classic shapes – from totes and shoppers to bowling and hobo bags – in leather or the traditional Burberry check. The iconic check is updated in different colours, including the black, white and grey of the Beat check, or the traditional House check, which sits beside the smaller-scale plaid of the Haymarket check. All are combined with leather trims, handles and details.

With two Royal Warrants and a unique history that spans three centuries, Burberry is ingrained in British heritage, synonymous with quality and British style, and is exported to all corners of the globe.

OPPOSITE Metallic leather tile tote.

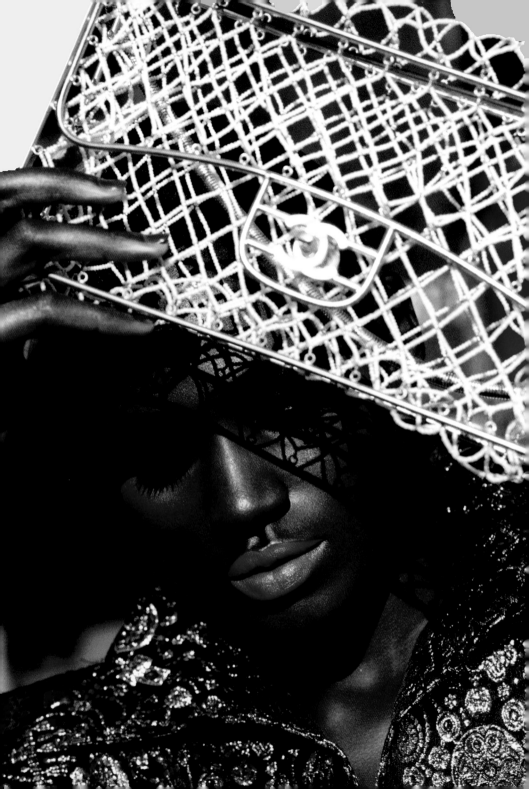

CHANEL

CHANEL epitomizes French style, with
designs that are as classic as they are
modern and as luxurious as they are
crafted. Home to the revolutionary 2.55,
possibly the most famous handbag in the
world, the label and the bag are as
desirable today as they ever were.

OPPOSITE Net bag, CHANEL Ready-to-Wear Collection
S/S 97.

Founded in 1909
www.chanel.com

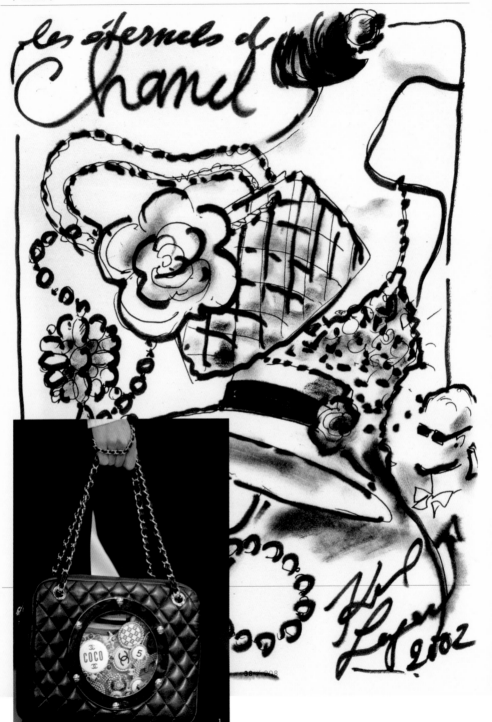

TRULY AN ENDURING CLASSIC, CHANEL'S 2.55 BAG HAS BEEN REINVENTED IN EVERYTHING FROM DENIM AND TWEED TO TERRY TOWELING.

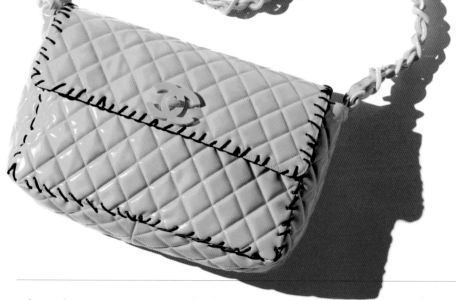

1 U-Boat bag, CHANEL Ready-to-Wear Collection S/S 08.
2 Karl Lagerfeld sketch, Les éternels de CHANEL 2002.
3 The 2.55 quilted bag in neon yellow.

In February 1955 a fashion legend was born. With its distinctive quilted black lambskin and gold-chain strap, the CHANEL 2.55 bag has become one of the most covetable and instantly recognizable bags in fashion history – a modern design classic. It has inspired every CHANEL bag since its creation, as well as many imitations, but nothing comes close to the real thing.

One of the world's biggest fashion brands, CHANEL is synonymous with luxury and style. Creator Gabrielle Chanel was a pioneering force in fashion during the first half of the twentieth century, revolutionizing the way women dressed. She put women in trousers, invented the 'little black dress', introduced costume jewellery to high fashion and her signature perfume CHANEL No˙5 was the first perfume to take the name of a designer.

Chanel enjoyed numerous groundbreaking achievements in the world of design, but none so much as the bag she released in February 1955, a design classic that has withstood the test of time. The 2.55, named for the date it was launched, is the design house's signature bag. Distinctive in style – a rectangular-shaped black lambskin quilted box, with chain strap – its simplicity and elegance belies the history behind it. The later Classic version features the famous interlinked double-Cs logo on the clasp.

When the bag was launched it caused a sensation. Traditionally women's bags had been handheld which, in 1955, was cumbersome and no longer practical for modern women busy with family lives, work and travel. Chanel was quoted as saying that she

'was fed up with holding my purses in my hands and losing them, so I added a strap and carried them over my shoulder'.

By adding a shoulder strap, previously reserved for soldiers' and bikers' bags, she revolutionized the way women carried bags – and held themselves.

The signature quilting on the bag, now an intrinsic part of the brand's heritage, was inspired both by stable boys' coats as well as Gabrielle Chanel's own cushions from the sofa of her Rue Cambon apartment in Paris.

As beautifully crafted today as they were in 1955, it takes the brand's atelier more than 180 product stages to create a 2.55 bag. As much attention to detail is paid to the inside of the bag as to the outside. Lined in claret red and including secret pockets as well as a lipstick pocket, the 2.55 is a place to keep your secrets as well as belongings. Far from the IT bags that are popular for one season, this iconic bag transcends fashion-fickle trends, proving to be just as covetable now as it was 50 years ago. Indeed, over 30 new models are produced each year, forming an integral part of the design house's eight annual collections.

All of the CHANEL bags designed since the 2.55 have been inspired by the original. Creative Director Karl Lagerfeld plays with the house's signature motifs to produce bags that are witty, modern and highly desirable – but always instantly recognizable as CHANEL. Many of them share characteristics such as quilting, chain straps and use of logo, updated in different shapes and fabrics.

In January 2008 CHANEL debuted its most luxurious and expensive bag yet, the White Alligator and Diamonds 2.55. Made from white alligator skin and featuring the double-C clasp in 18-carat white gold encrusted with over 300 3.56-carat diamonds, only 13 bags were available worldwide, making it possibly the most exclusive – as well as luxurious – 2.55 ever made.

While some versions of the bags have been slightly tongue-in-cheek, such as the black and white Hat bag from 1988 or the extra-long Baguette bag from 1990, others remain true to the brand's ethos of luxury, craftsmanship and quality.

Today the classic black 2.55, once a favourite of style icons such as Jackie Kennedy and Brigitte Bardot, has found resonance with a new generation of stylish young women. Kate Moss is reported to own over 100 CHANEL bags, while other modern style icons such as Chloe Sevigny, Mary-Kate Olsen, Sarah Jessica Parker, Sienna Miller, Keira Knightley and Kirsten Dunst have all been photographed carrying them.

The 2.55 perfectly encapsulates CHANEL's appeal. It crosses generations – whether you are sixteen or sixty it appears elegant and youthful, sophisticated and stylish – making it a truly timeless design classic.

OPPOSITE 1 CHANEL 2.55 Exotics, 2008. 2 Quilted bag, CHANEL Ready-to-Wear Collection A/W 09/10. 3 Small black leather shopping bag, CHANEL Ready-to-Wear Collection, S/S 09.

OVER THE PAGE
(Left) New edition of the 2.55 bag in black aged leather. (Right) Clutch in black quilted leather and white tweed with two-tone camellias, pearls and sequins, CHANEL Ready-to-Wear Collection S/S 01.

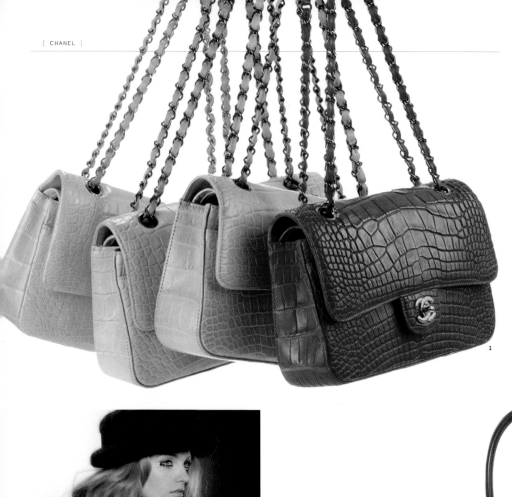

1

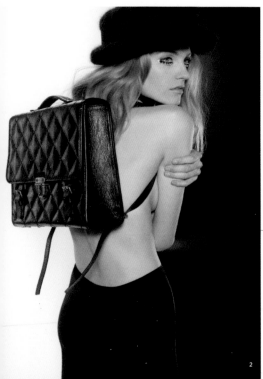

41 / 208

2

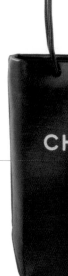

CHA

3

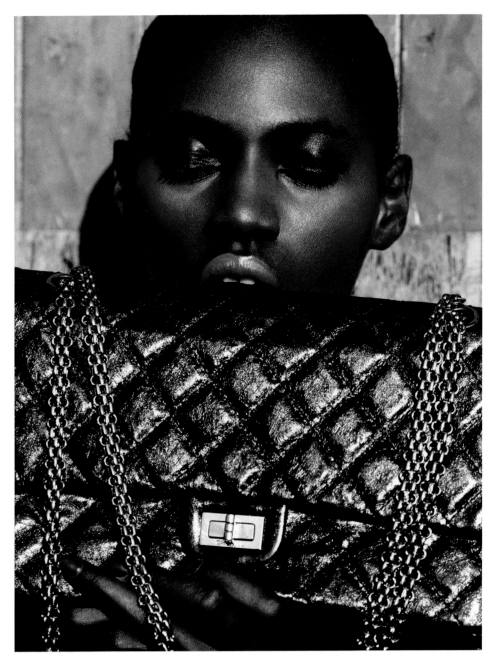

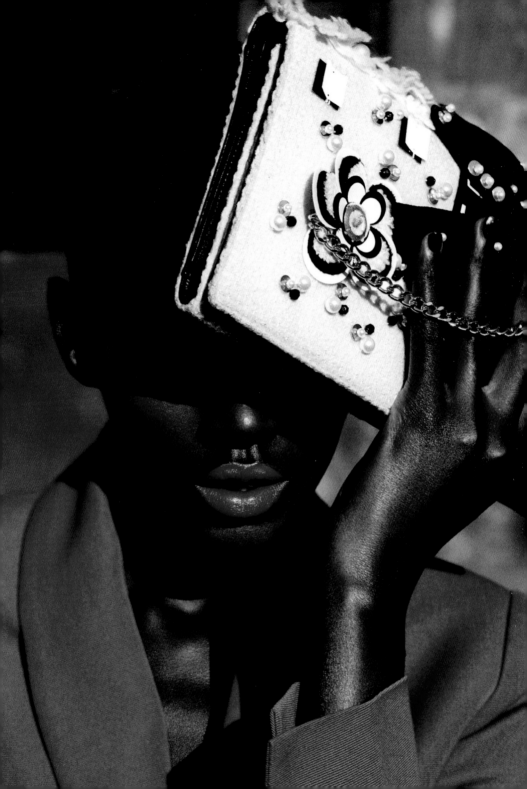

CHARLOTT VASBERG

Charlott Vasberg bags consist of softly draped shapes that combine the structured with the fluid, the hard with the soft, always with an emphasis on functional hardware and signature zip detailing.

OPPOSITE Designer's sketches writ large in Beijing's Forbidden City.

Founded in 2004
www.charlottvasberg.com

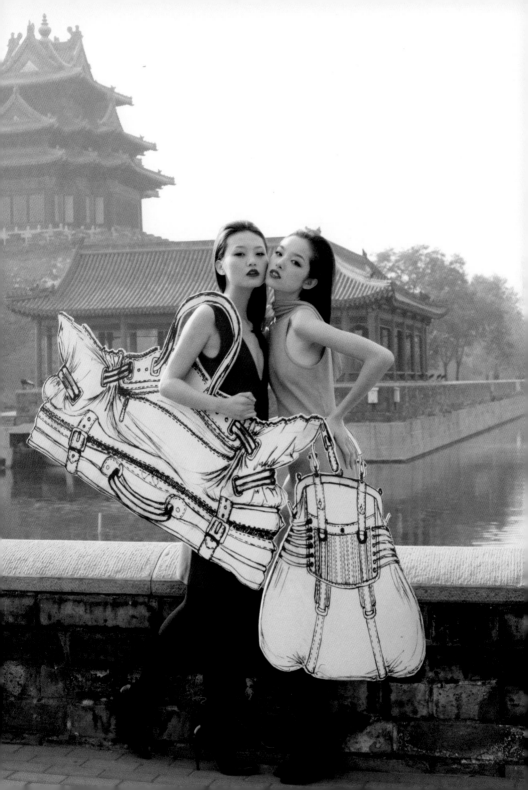

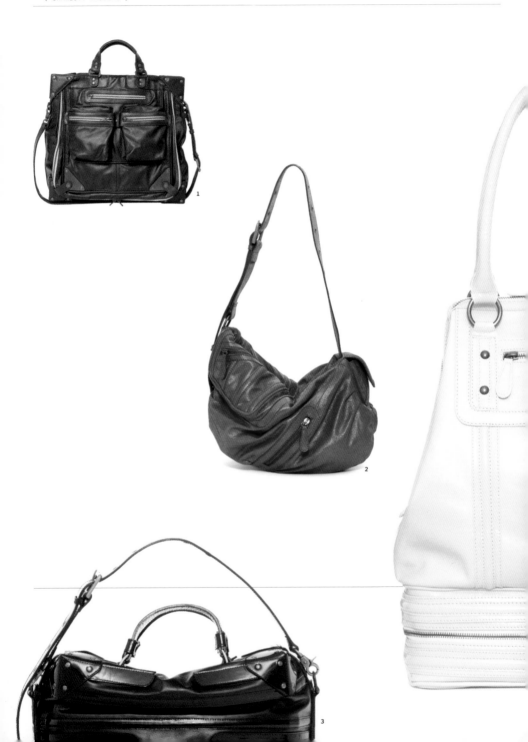

1

2

3

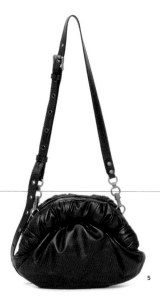

'DRAPING USING UNUSUAL TRIMMINGS AND COMBINING TRADITIONAL CRAFT TECHNIQUES WITH MODERN SHAPES AND DETAILING IS MY SIGNATURE DESIGN STYLE'

6

1 Pocket Suitcase Shopper in midnight blue, S/S 08.
2 Pocket Bag in Red Sunday. 3 Black Suitcase Bag, S/S 09.
4 White-mix CV Shopper 5 Midnight blue small Circle Bag.
6 Thick Buckle Belt bag, S/S 08.

4

5

A womenswear graduate turned accessories designer, Swedish-born Charlott Vasberg applies her knowledge of garment construction to bags, and is focused on creating beautiful and original designs. Vasberg has said that in the future she hopes that

'customers will become less interested in celebrity endorsed products and yearn to be individual once again.'

Consumers could do a lot worse than invest in a bag from Charlott Vasberg, whose unique designs mix strong functional elements with a subtle feminine sensibility.

The four-year-old label started after Vasberg finished her Womenswear MA at London's Central Saint Martins. This apparel design background has continued to influence the way she works, from ruched shapes to the use of garment details and trimmings:

'I have always loved bags and accessories and thought it would be a good way to begin',

she says.

Inspired by unusual items, random ideas and her own archive of accessories, the designer works three-dimensionally, using leather to recreate ideas inspired by experimentation with drapes and detailing.

'Draping using unusual trimmings and combining traditional craft techniques with modern shapes and detailing is my signature design style',

Vasberg explains.

Vasberg creates modern draped shapes by applying her apparel designer's approach to accessories. This otherwise unusual approach to bag design has proved to be very successful. Vasberg's fluid, versatile shapes combine with zips and metal hardware detailing to create soft feminine designs with tough undertones. Working with leather, Vasberg is also known for inverting traditional styles – a hard shape will become a soft style, and vice versa. Unusual detailing such as secret compartments and zip-off bases are also key features, while multiple signature zip detailing add a quirky touch. Trimmings also influence the bag styles, from zips and press studs to signature designs for trimmings and bag frames.

The bag Vasberg is most recognized for is the Ziprow twist bag from her first collection, which is distinctive for its use of decorative zips. Other signature pieces include the Draped Suitcase Bag, which takes inspiration from vintage luggage and mixes it with multiple zips both decorative and functional, and the Old School Bag, which updates a classic satchel style into a sexy and slouchy over-the-shoulder bag with purse-pocket detailing.

For Spring/Summer 09 the designer took inspiration from forms and silhouettes, using fluid shapes with elements of corsetry construction to create pieces that are structured yet delicate at the same time. As usual, shapes are versatile, with different carrying options and functional outside-pocket detailing that allow the bag to be divided into sections. Key shapes range from asymmetric forms to clutches with geometric detailing. The colour palette of pastel tones, including soft peach, patent blue and sun-blushed almond, sit alongside patent base colours of black and white, and the darker metallic bronze and pewter.

Spring/Summer 09 also saw the debut of a new line for the brand called 'Re-collections'. The styles are a reflection of the classic Charlott Vasberg shapes, but use playful prints and cotton canvases, with leather detailing highlights.

Shape and detailing are the focus for Vasberg's Autumn/Winter 09/10 collection, with Art Deco architecture subtly referenced in the use of geometric features. Soft, padded sections are balanced with defined angular lines, while smooth curved shapes feature asymmetric draping and structured panels. Styles range from classic oversized clutches to modern reinvented doctor bags and intricately detailed soft frame bags.

Bought exclusively for Selfridges when it first debuted, the label is now sold internationally in major high-end department stores and boutiques, and its reputation and fan base continues to grow.

OPPOSITE Designer's sketches.

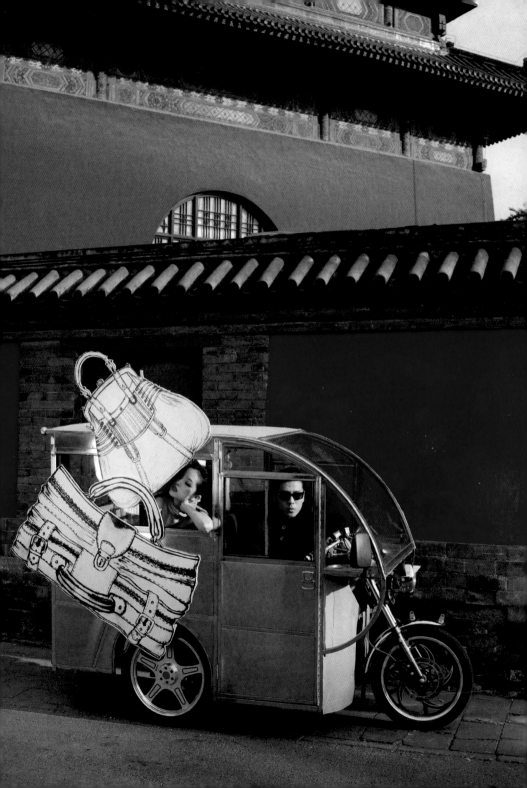

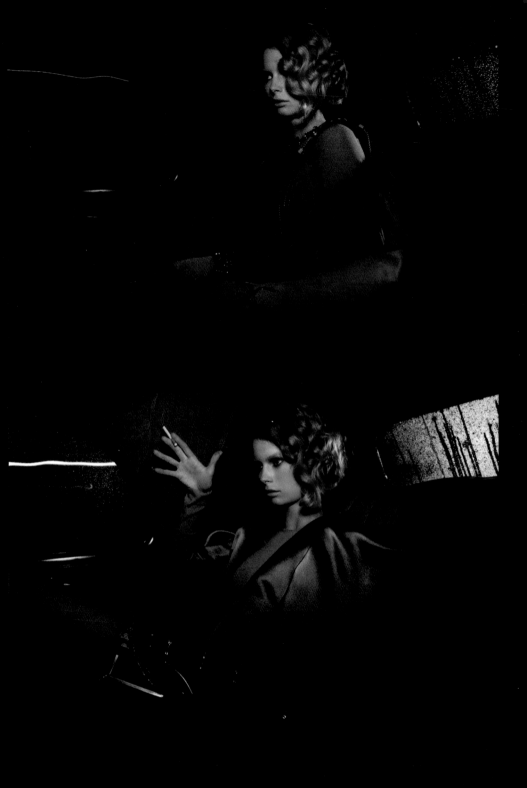

CHLOÉ

With its nonchalant French style and an accessories
line filled with hit bags — from the must-have
Paddington to the Bay bag and the Paraty — Chloé is
one of the most desired brands in the world.

OPPOSITE (top) Heloise in cream leather with chain
detail; (below) Pochette in noir.

Founded in 1952
www.chloe.com

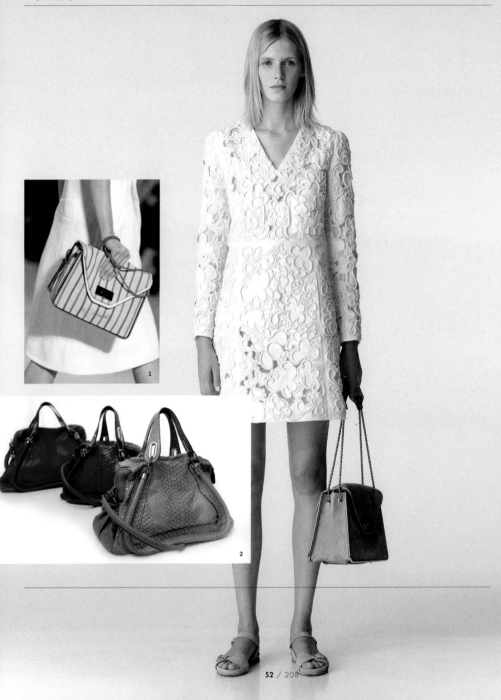

1

2

3

THE ROMANTIC AND ULTRA FEMININE CHLOÉ LOOK HAS COME TO DEFINE COOL FOR A GENERATION OF YOUNG WOMEN

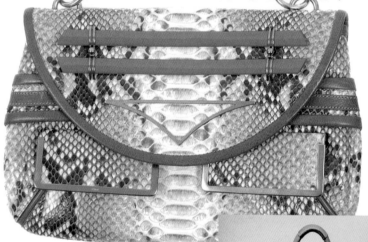

1 Striped canvas Sally bag, S/S 09. 2 Paraty bags, A/W 09/10. 3 Sally bag, S/S 09. 4 Paddington bag, S/S 05. 5 Irini bag, A/W 08/09.

4

5

Although over 50 years old, French fashion house Chloé is one of the few luxury brands that retains a youthful spirit. Popular with an international young clientele wanting to buy into the brand's pretty and feminine aesthetic, Chloé is one of those rare labels. It doesn't try to be cool, it just is.

Founded in 1952 by Egyptian-born Parisienne Gaby Aghion, the Chloé identity has always been tied up with moving against the grain. Rejecting the stiff formality of 1950s fashion, the label created soft, body-conscious clothes from fine fabrics. This helped set the tone for the romantic clothes that came to epitomize youthful and modern design – hallmarks which continue to this day.

Hiring new talent to design the collections has become part of the Chloé legacy, starting with Karl Lagerfeld, who took the post of Head Designer in 1966. Under his direction, the label became one of the most iconic fashion brands of the 1970s. Chloé's romantic designs reflected that decade's glamorous hippie aesthetic perfectly, and helped define the look of a generation. It also attracted high-profile fans, including Jackie Kennedy, Bridget Bardot, Maria Callas and Grace Kelly.

In recent years Stella McCartney's appointment worked in the brand's favour, bringing it both publicity as well as a certain 'London girl' cool. Together with Phoebe Philo, who later took over the creative direction, McCartney helped propel the brand to new levels of success and played a key role in making it a must-have label for a new generation of young women.

While Chloé's floaty, feminine designs have proved to be highly desirable, the brand's accessory line is equally – if not more – covetable. Consistently producing glamorous arm candy for girls about town, the label became a household name thanks to the massive popularity of the Paddington bag.

Undoubtedly the brand's biggest hit, this slouchy, unstructured soft leather bag with trademark oversized lock and key bearing the Chloé logo, was launched in 2005 to runaway success. The hype surrounding the Paddington bag was so great that it sold out before it had even arrived in the shops, causing a sensation. Copycat designs and fakes quickly flooded the market. The influence of the Paddington can still be seen in bag design, from the slouchy shape to the giant lock detail. The label updates this classic every season by introducing different colourways and fabrications, as well as offering variations inspired by the original.

Although Chloé hasn't produced another IT bag on the scale of the Paddington, it has continued to design gorgeous, retro-tinged leather bags that are highly sought after. For Spring/Summer 06 the label had a hit with the Edith bag, whose design was likened to that of a casual Kelly bag. Made in leather with little detailing except for the obvious contrast stitching, the clean lines of the Edith design create an authentic 1970s feel.

The Bay bag from Spring/Summer 07 is another key piece from the Chloé archive. More retro looking, it features a quilted front and three zipped compartments. Oversized leather zip pullers are a key characteristic of the bag.

For Autumn/Winter 08/09 Chloé's bags became more decorative and graphic, mixing bold jewel colours with contrast animal skin and metal hardware trims. The must-have from this collection is the Paraty bag, which comes in two versions: a vegetal calfskin or a more exclusive slightly shiny python. Shapes include a shopper, a tote and a flat shoulder bag version. With minimal hardware and rolled leather detailing, the Paraty is both sexy and sophisticated and very, very desirable. Much like the Chloé brand itself.

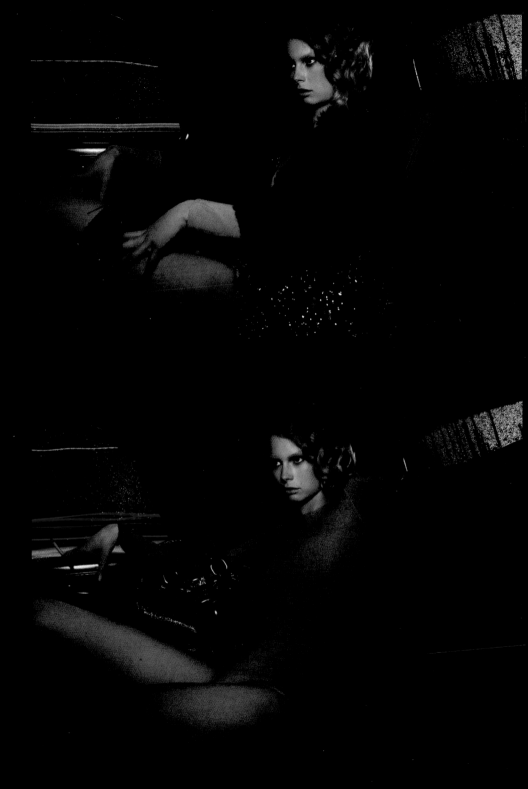

CORTO MOLTEDO

Corto Moltedo redefines the traditional ideals of luxury. Reflecting the designer's own heritage, the brand represents a unique blend of pop-luxe that combines classic Italian style with cutting-edge New York chic.

OPPOSITE Priscilla Rocket shoulder bag, A/W 08/09.

Founded in 2004
www.corto.com

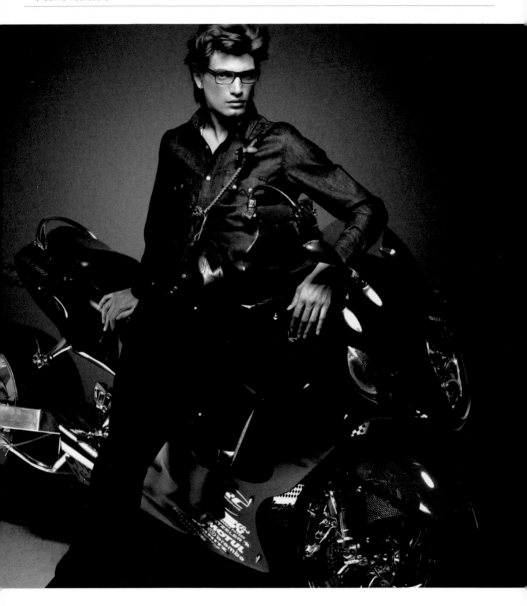

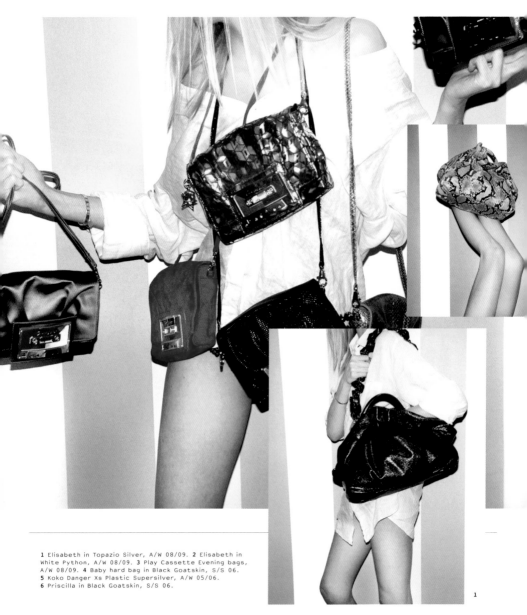

1 Elisabeth in Topazio Silver, A/W 08/09. 2 Elisabeth in
White Python, A/W 08/09. 3 Play Cassette Evening bags,
A/W 08/09. 4 Baby hard bag in Black Goatskin, S/S 06.
5 Koko Danger Xs Plastic Supersilver, A/W 05/06.
6 Priscilla in Black Goatskin, S/S 06.

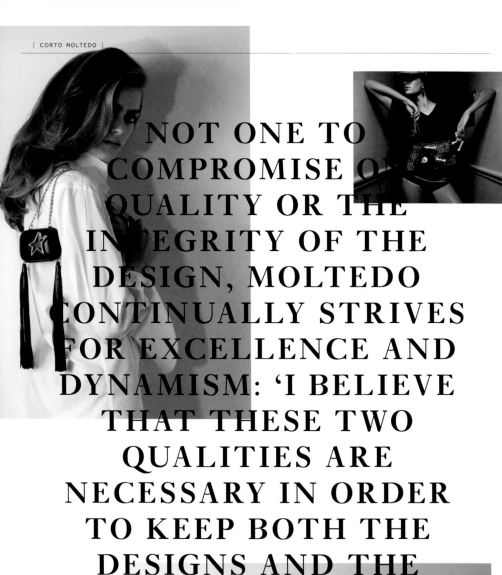

NOT ONE TO COMPROMISE ON QUALITY OR THE INTEGRITY OF THE DESIGN, MOLTEDO CONTINUALLY STRIVES FOR EXCELLENCE AND DYNAMISM: 'I BELIEVE THAT THESE TWO QUALITIES ARE NECESSARY IN ORDER TO KEEP BOTH THE DESIGNS AND THE BRAND IMAGE FRESH.'

The visionary behind the brand, Gabrielecorto Moltedo designs from his base in Paris and his research and development studio in Florence.

Born and raised in New York City, Gabrielecorto Moltedo has been immersed in the fashion world from a very young age. His parents, Laura and Vittorio Moltedo, founded the Italian luxury label Bottega Veneta, and Moltedo frequently accompanied them on their travels, absorbing their passion, artistry and commitment to creating quality products with global appeal:

'Because it was in the family, working in fashion has always made sense to me.'

Several summers working in the family factory in the Venetian countryside exposed Moltedo to the intricacies of traditional Italian leather craftsmanship. It was during this period that Moltedo came to comprehend the detail required for conceiving and executing a truly stunning design. After graduating from New York University, Moltedo earned a Master's degree from Emerson College before creating his own label.

Moltedo has always been surrounded by a diverse range of cultural influences:

'I consider myself a multicultural person, I have some very distinctive New York influences that I try to merge with those from my Italian heritage. I can't picture myself having to choose between the two, so I strive to bring out the best of both in my collections'.

He therefore merges the dynamism and edginess of New York with the traditional shapes, colours, materials and forms of the Italian and French style.

Moltedo's designs never lose sight of the people he is creating for:

'I always bear in mind my friends, their lives, their needs and their style when preparing a new line'.

The designer is drawn to people who dare to make fashion statements, such as Madonna, Julianne Moore and Devon Aoki. Moltedo considers Charlotte Dellal, sister of model and DJ Alice Dellal, as the epitome of the Corto Moltedo woman's style. He has come to think of her as his muse:

'Classy, elegant and well-travelled; her style resembles her personality, making her undeniably original.'

Attracting widespread recognition following their launch, Moltedo's signature styles include the Priscilla Bag, acclaimed for its innovative form as a shoulder bag, and the Susan Clutch, praised for its refined chic and practicality. The M-Dolla Clutch was designed specifically to suit Madonna's needs on her world tour, and has enjoyed worldwide publicity.

Moltedo draws heavily on the art world when he's researching a collection,

'I have always admired the work of architect Tadao Ando, minimalist and deconstructionist … In military museums I can often draw ideas from looking at the design and cuts of naval and infantry uniforms'.

Though Moltedo maintains that his biggest influences remain the distinct styles of each of his parents, the Corto Moltedo vision is inimitably and unmistakably his own.

This unique vision is also evident in the designer's choice of branding. When researching his very first collection he saw the need to come up with something distinctive that would make the brand instantly recognizable, and he decided upon his initial 'C' together with a star. Moltedo saw the star as a symbol of beauty but also subconsciously associated in the West with military power, the perfect representation of modern women – beautiful and chic yet strong and dynamic.

Never without his trusty moleskin notebook, Moltedo is forever sketching,

'I design all the time, whether that be in my offices in Paris or Florence, in the street, at a café or a museum',

he explains. Back in the studio, the designer then begins the long yet exhilarating process of transforming his sketches – choosing fabrics and materials and trialing prototypes until he is satisfied that he has created the bag he originally envisioned. While this is a long process, Moltedo sees it as necessary in order to keep the brand and the designs fresh as he continually strives for excellence.

OPPOSITE Susan Skeptic, A/W 08/09.

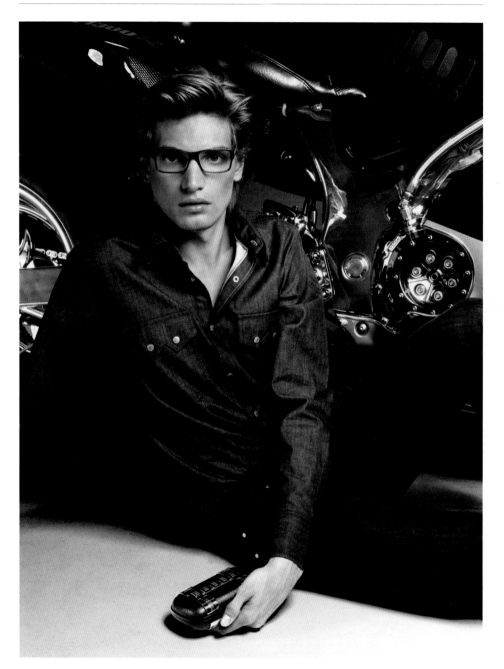

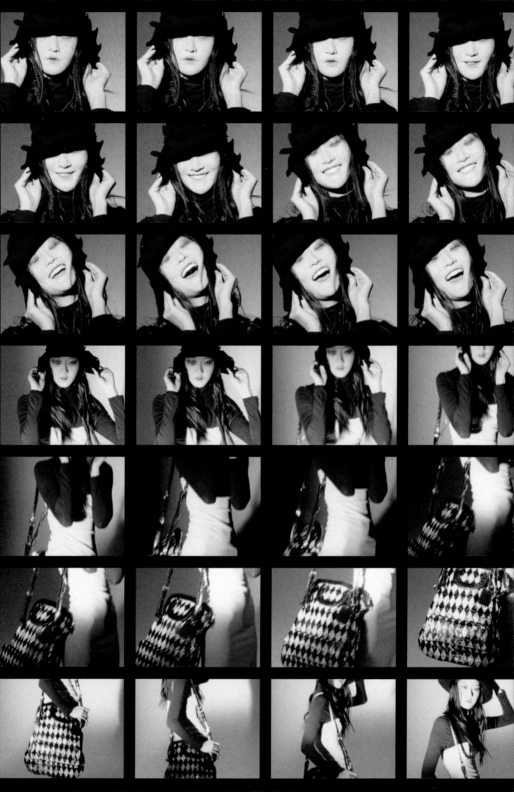

DOLCE
&
GABBANA

Renowned for their supremely sexy and beautiful designs, Dolce&Gabbana is a global household name, exporting the glamour of Italy to the rest of the world.

OPPOSITE Miss Pocket, S/S 08 collection.

Founded in 1985
www.dolcegabbana.it

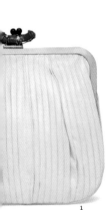

1

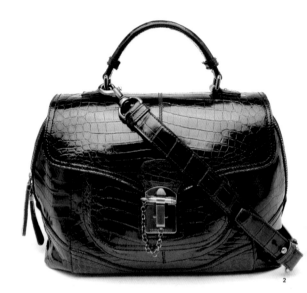

2

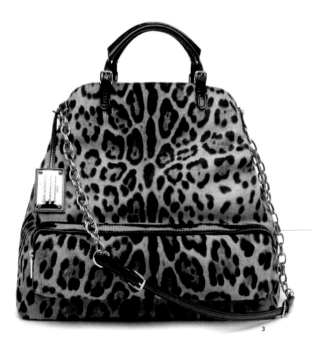

3

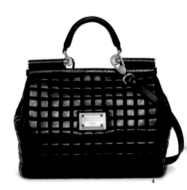

4

BY OFFERING EXCLUSIVE PIECES AS WELL AS READY-TO-WEAR COLLECTIONS, DOLCE&GABBANA CONTINUE TO CREATE A LUXURY BRAND THAT WILL STAND THE TEST OF TIME.

1 Miss Katharine, A/W 09/10. 2 Miss Catch, A/W 08/09.
3 Miss Pocket, A/W 07/08. 4 Miss Sicily, A/W 09/10. 5 Miss
Easy Way, S/S 08, Limited Edition. 6 Miss Charles, S/S 09.
7 Miss Pocket, S/S 08.

Given their influence in the fashion industry, it's hard to believe that Italian luxury brand Dolce&Gabbana has only been established for just over 20 years. Starting with a women's line in 1985, the label has expanded at a fast pace and now encompasses menswear, the younger 'D&G' line, accessories, eyewear, perfumes, children's line 'D&G Junior' and cosmetics – an impressive range by any brand's standard.

Domenico Dolce and Stefano Gabbana are the design duo behind Dolce&Gabbana, one of Italy's premier luxury brands. The pair met in the early 1980s when working as design assistants in Milan, and presented their first collection under the Dolce&Gabbana label in 1985 at a Milan fashion show celebrating new talent. They quickly established themselves as noteworthy young designers and built their brand steadily, adding menswear, perfume, lingerie and accessories, as well as the 'D&G' line, in 1994.

Their designs celebrate the female form and take inspiration from the strong, stylish women of their native Italy. As such, Dolce&Gabbana has long been a red carpet favourite with celebrities – the highly glamorous and sexy clothes have dressed much of Hollywood, along with high profile music stars and style icons. Indeed, Dolce&Gabbana features in Madonna's stable of select designers, exclusively designing 1,500 costumes for her Girlie Tour in 1993, and dressing the star for the launch of her Music album in 2000. They also exclusively dressed pop princess Kylie Minogue for her 2002 Fever world tour and provided clothes and accessories for Whitney Houston's world tour in 1999.

This association with celebrity, coupled with the designers' ability to turn their hands to any aspect of design has helped propel Dolce&Gabbana into a highly regarded, globally recognized brand in a very short space of time.

Accessories form a key part of each Dolce&Gabbana collection and take inspiration from the main clothing line. The designers returned to their roots when designing the Spring/Summer 09 range, which is influenced by Sicily and the richness of the Baroque period. Entitled 'Baroque Pyjama', the range focused on menswear pyjama shapes and luxe fabrics. This innovative approach translated into heavily embellished and decorated pieces for the bag line, which also makes use of precious materials such as brooches, pearls and gold chains. Featuring rectangular pochettes and envelope

bags in glove leather, suede and nappa mordoré, padded nappa and raw-edged mignon, the designs are embellished with double-faced sequins or mirrored leather mosaic. These highly decorated pieces contrast with simple, structured shapes from the Miss Sicily line (from the same collection), which features more serious and austere designs inspired by the elegance of women from the south of Italy.

Must-have bags from the brand include the versatile Miss Easy Way. It has been presented in many collections, in a variety of sizes, including mini versions, and in materials ranging from soft leather to laminated and embroidered leather, and in a wide range of colours.

The covetable Miss Pocket, Autumn/Winter 07/08, was created in laminated python, laminated layers, suede and patent. Designed as a day bag but closer in style to an oversized travel bag, it has a maxi pocket that ideally zips off to create another bag entirely, making it a multi-functional yet super-luxurious style.

Bags that have a dual function reappear throughout the brand's accessories collections, but this feature does not come at the expense of luxury and good craftsmanship. Artisan touches such as layers of snakeskin, multi-coloured mosaic patchwork, colour blocked leathers and delicate silk tulle wrapped over brocade or leather to resemble a veil ensure that Dolce&Gabbana bags are as beautiful as they are practical. In 2006 the label introduced a new line of accessories called 'Animalier', which makes heavy use of the leopard print that has become one of the signatures of the brand. The following year they presented their first collection of crocodile travel cases for men. Every coveted piece in the collection is custom made and features unique details.

Continuing the theme of luxury and exclusivity, in 2008 Dolce&Gabbana launched a range of limited-edition bags made from exotic skins, including crocodile and python. Consisting of classic, hallmark Dolce&Gabbana shapes with interesting twists, the range also introduced new shapes such as the Lounge bag, a petite shoulder bag with signature details such as an exterior zip pocket. Also new was the elongated satchel with shoulder strap that, when folded, creates a maxi clutch. Only ten of each style in the range was produced, making it a truly unique collection.

MAIN PICTURE Miss Sicily, A/W 09/10.
INSET Miss Katharine, A/W 09/10.
OVER THE PAGE Miss Charles, S/S 09.

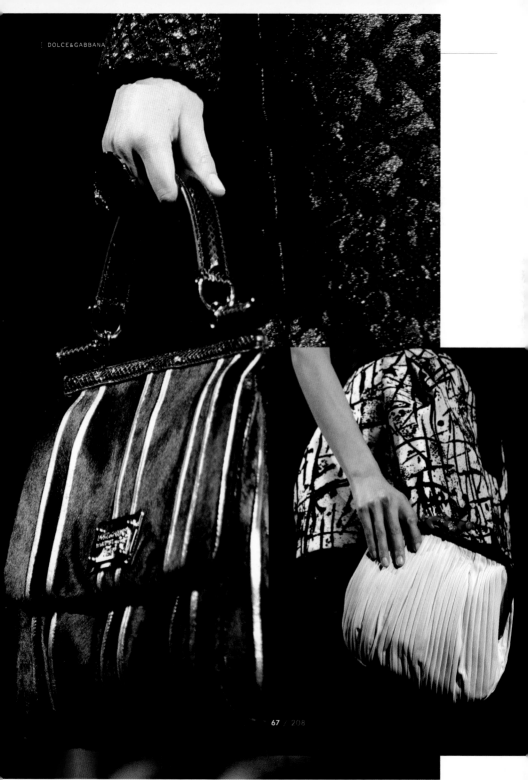

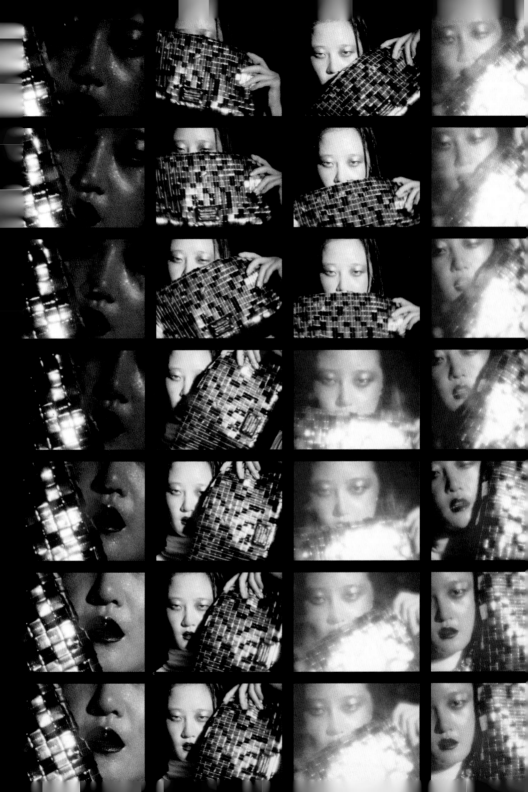

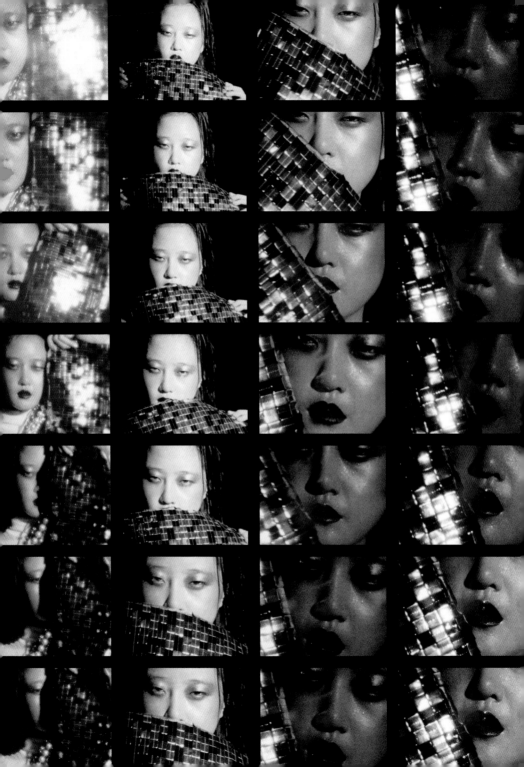

Reacting against the overexposure of mass produced bags, Erva sets out to create uniquely flirtatious and delicious bags that have a touch of humour.

ERVA

OPPOSITE B.31 Box Clutch, A/W 08/09.

Founded in 2001
www.erva-design.com

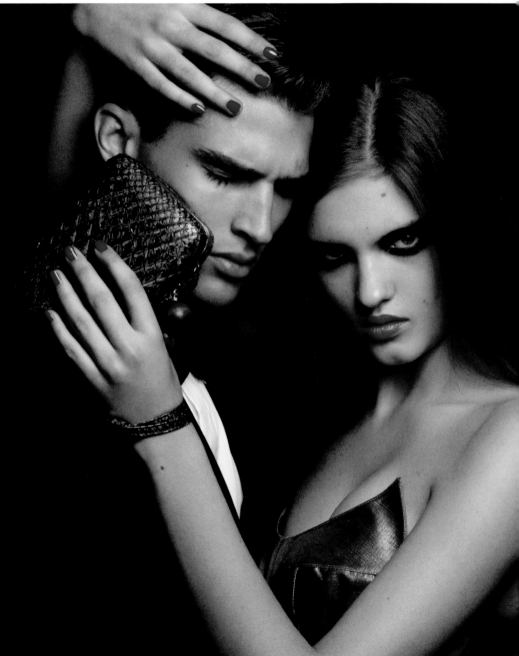

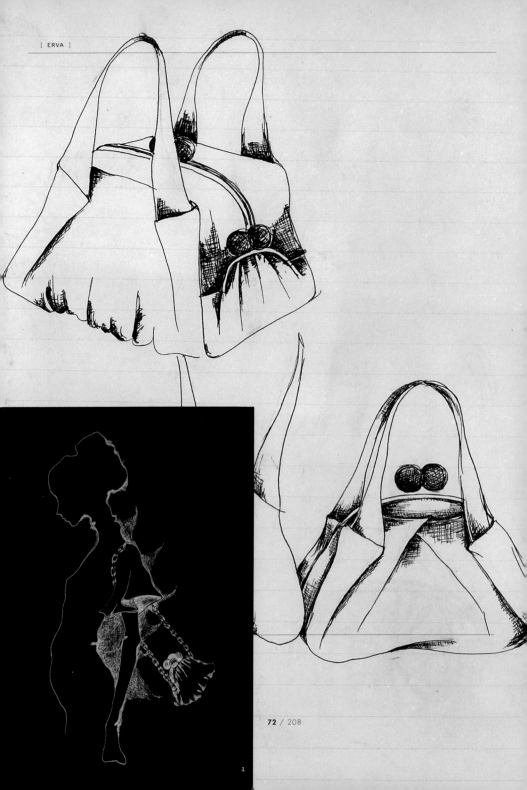

'OUR BAGS ARE REALLY PIECES OF CRAFTSMANSHIP, EVERYTHING IS CUT AND ASSEMBLED BY HAND, TECHNOLOGY HASN'T ARRIVED IN OUR FACTORY YET'

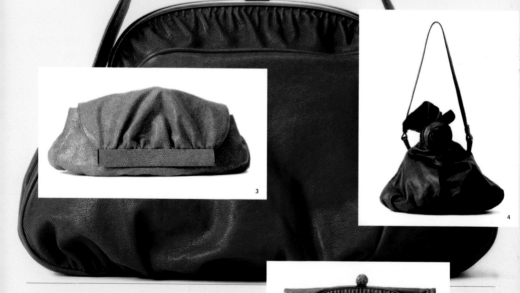

1 Design sketch in chalk. 2 Designer's sketchbook.
3 M.855, 40s clutch, A/W 08/09. 4 M.865, Garter, A/W
08/09. 5 M.802, Ninotska L, A/W 08/09. 6 M.815, Shell,
A/W 08/09.

Already making waves among the fashion savvy, Erva is the creation of two complementary personalities, Eva García and Rosa Rial, who met when they were both working as designers in Spain. The pair have now been designing for over eight years, and refer to themselves simply as 'bag makers'. They make a point of not responding to fast-paced fashion trends, choosing instead to design bags without logos or overtly fussy hardware in the hope of creating bags that have a personal, timeless quality.

'The IT bag fever and logo-mania is overexploited' explains García, who also speculates that in the future – and particularly in the digital era – people will be more receptive to simple and lasting beauty; forsaking quantity for quality in their consumer habits.

Eva García and Rosa Rial met while designing ready-to-wear accessories in Spain. They moved to London shortly afterwards, where they decided to start designing their own collection:

'We realized that it was difficult to find bags we loved, at the time there weren't many young designers doing bags in leather and we wanted to buy anonymous pieces in fine leathers with a unique style.'

Erva bags possess this unique style, and are not only stocked in some of the world's most prestigious stores but have become a coveted brand that is synonymous with both cutting-edge trendsetters and some of the world's most stylish celebrities. Lou Doillon, the model and actress daughter of Jane Birkin, the Olsen twins and Cameron Diaz are all fans of the brand and have been photographed sporting Erva bags on numerous Hollywood outings.

Inspired by the minutiae of their everyday surroundings, the designers reveal that they don't have a particular method when designing: García insists,

'The truth is that there is no process, we don't usually have a theme – or at least it is not intentional – we respond to impulses and desires. Rosa is more creative and I am more practical, yet luckily for us we complement each other and always agree on the look that we want.'

This serendipitous designing method is one of Erva's trademarks. Whether it's a material or a piece of hardware, intuition always guides the creative process:

'The first collection came with the discovery of frames from the 1940s. We love the retro style frames give but then try to change it into something more modern'.

While the designers use no visible branding, their designs speak for themselves: instantly recognizable for the use of their wooden-pip frame closures, which feature on the majority of their bags, both as a main closure and, more interestingly, as an external pocket closure. The Box Clutch is also a unique Erva style that many customers identify with the brand.

Erva's collections are predominantly made in leather, a material the designers simultaneously love for its tactile qualities and the way it ages, and yet find challenging. Working mainly with soft leathers to create their signature detailing, the duo use only the best quality smooth and textured hides and incorporate some exotic skins to add depth. Beautifully handcrafted features include such details as pleats, ruffles, twists and flowers.

The designers' dedication to cutting, workmanship and finishing touches have become synonymous with the Erva aesthetic. As for the future, the pair consider themselves lucky to own their growing workshop and still directly manage and influence the production of their increasingly sought-after designs, enabling them to retain the unique qualities and look of the brand that they have worked so hard to achieve.

OPPOSITE Wallet, S/S 08.

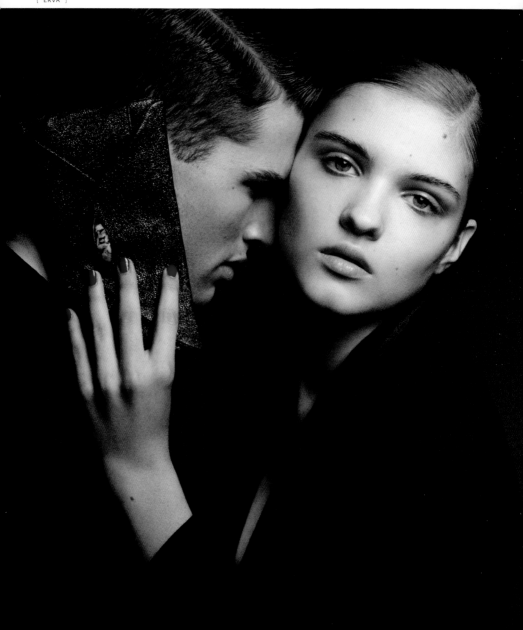

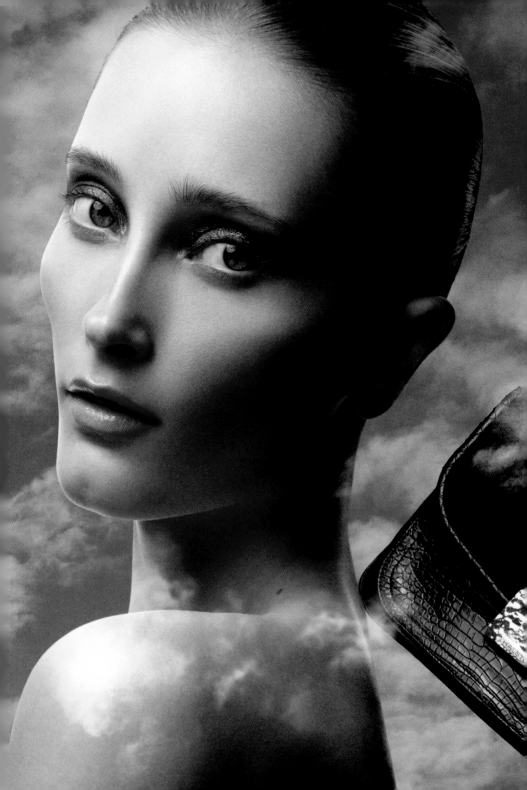

One of America's greatest designers,
Halston originally found fame in the disco
era of the 1970s. Newly relaunched, the
brand celebrates the designer's aesthetic
of simplicity, elegance and luxury and gives
it a modern perspective.

HALSTON

OPPOSITE Liz convertible clutch in black crocodile
and suede, A/W 08/09.

Founded in 1968
www.halston.com

Roy Halston Frowick found initial fame and success as a milliner, creating the pillbox hat that Jackie Kennedy made famous, before moving on to design the women's ready-to-wear fashion that would ensure his place in fashion history. Famous for his ultrasuede shirtdress and fluid jersey pieces, he attracted a high-profile celebrity fan base who fell in love with the glamour, clean lines and simplicity of his designs. The Halston name and design ethos has been relaunched as a luxury 21st century brand for a new generation.

Halston's heyday was undoubtedly the 1970s, the decade, some say, that taste forgot. Not Halston, however. When others around him were showcasing elaborate and fussy designs, he created simple and luxurious garments that focused on cut, fabric and colour. The result was elegant and chic separates and dresses that were perfectly in tune and at home in the glamorous Studio 54 disco era of the late 1970s. The name Halston had become synonymous with American style. *Newsweek* named him the 'premier fashion designer of all America' and he counted celebrities including Liza Minelli, Andy Warhol and Bianca Jagger as friends as well as clients.

The new Halston pays homage to its founder and iconic designer, respecting his design aesthetics of simplicity, elegance and luxury, but adding a modern interpretation. The brand's bag line follows the same design principles as the clothing – clean and effortless designs that focus on shape and fabric with a hint of metal detailing.

The label's goal is to capture a spirit of individuality while evading seasonal trends, creating designs that will suit each Halston girl – from the oversized clutch that makes the transition into a soft day bag to the chain-strap detail that adds edginess to a soft suede piece and the slouchy hobo bag that melds seamlessly with any aesthetic.

The brand has seen a shift away from the craze for one shape and size of bag for a given season to the search for designs that feel like one-of-a-kind. The notion of an IT bag has become redundant. Halston believes that the field of handbag design has become so diluted to a point that there are many variations – status bags, cool-factor bags and timeless classics.

Ultimately however, it's the quality of the fabrication and the focus on detail – from the discrete logo to the deceptively simple shapes and constructions – that makes a Halston bag special. Slouchy pochettes and envelope clutches in suedes, nappas and crocodile are all emblazoned with the signature Halston amulet in gold. The 'Halston Sac' in suede and leather from the Autumn/Winter 08/09 collection was dubbed the star bag of the season by UK *Vogue*. The easy daytime chic of the Sac also features in the Spring/Summer 09 collection, alongside super-luxe brilliant stone clutches.

The materials used in the bag range create a sense of depth, showcasing the brand's appreciation for the subtleties of skins in their most natural state. Simple shapes are transformed with highly saturated colours, or by adding fur trim in unexpected areas. Metal studs, crystal embellishments or the complete absence of enhancements, inform the mood of each collection from season to season.

The Autumn/Winter 09/10 range takes its cue from the mainline apparel collection, which is inspired by American style combined with a New York downtown attitude. Influenced by iconic 1980s female rock stars such as Debbie Harry, an edgy elegance sweeps through the collection, where New Wave meets luxury.

Ready-to-wear structures are reflected through the key bags – louche shapes in shoppers and iridescent python pouches. Anthracite metal hardware on straps and fastenings add a harder edge, while the Allen satchel contrasts suede and leather, alongside studding and snap Halston hardwear.

Although the Halston name has been famous for almost 50 years, in its current incarnation it is only a few seasons old and continues to grow. In July 2008 a stand-alone accessories boutique showcasing Halston handbags opened in the Room of Luxury at Harrods in London alongside brands such as Bottega Venetta, Marc Jacobs and Chloé, placing Halston strategically in the market while reinforcing the brand's dedication to developing its accessory line.

1 Maryse medium clutch in brown Zebra-printed ponyskin, S/S 09. 2 Foxy envelope clutch in bronze crinkle metallic, S/S 09. 3 Halston Sac in grey suede, A/W 08/09.

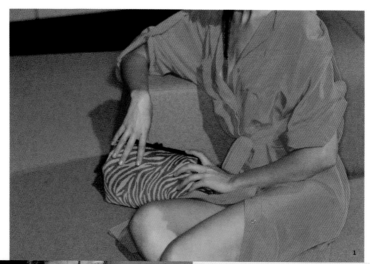

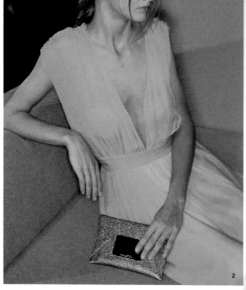

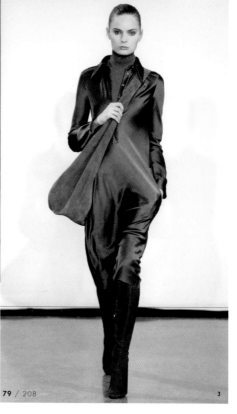

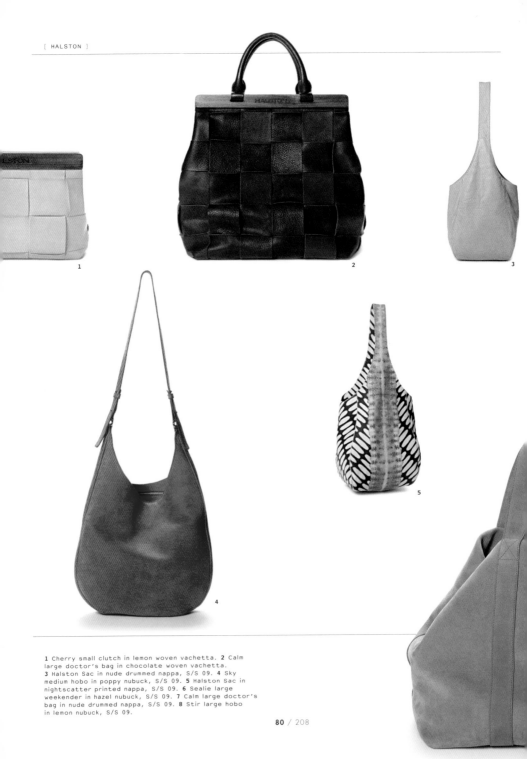

1 Cherry small clutch in lemon woven vachetta. 2 Calm
large doctor's bag in chocolate woven vachetta.
3 Halston Sac in nude drummed nappa, S/S 09. 4 Sky
medium hobo in poppy nubuck, S/S 09. 5 Halston Sac in
nightscatter printed nappa, S/S 09. 6 Sealie large
weekender in hazel nubuck, S/S 09. 7 Calm large doctor's
bag in nude drummed nappa, S/S 09. 8 Stir large hobo
in lemon nubuck, S/S 09.

SIMPLICITY OF DESIGN AND LUXURIOUS MATERIAL COMBINE TO CREATE THE UNCOMPLICATED YET LUXURIOUS BAGS THAT DO JUSTICE TO THE HALSTON NAME, ALL OVER AGAIN.

7

8

6

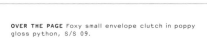

OVER THE PAGE Foxy small envelope clutch in poppy gloss python, S/S 09.

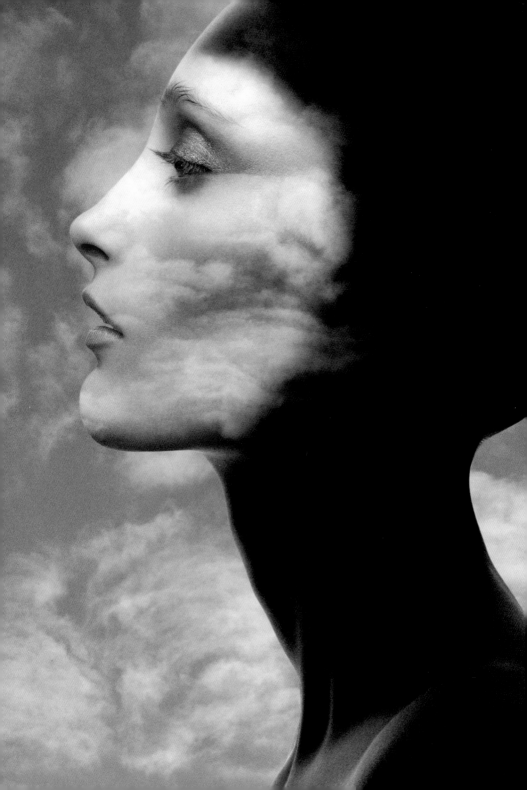

HERMÈS

One of the oldest and most covetable of brands, Hermès has created not one but two of the all-time classic bags with the Kelly and the Birkin. Exceptional craftsmanship, exquisite materials and attention to detail mean these heirloom bags never go out of style.

OPPOSITE (top) Red crocodile clutch; (below) Birkin bag in tan leather.

Founded in 1837
www.hermes.com

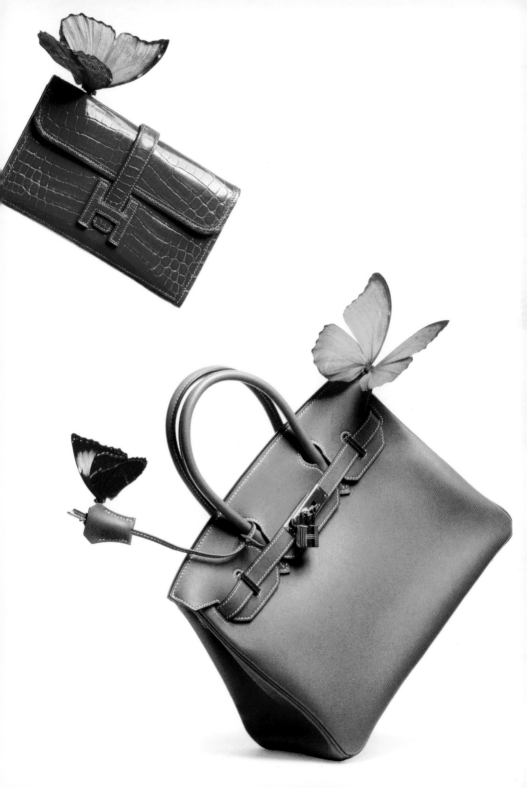

AN HERMÈS HANDBAG IS WIDELY CONSIDERED TO BE A WORK OF ART

—

THE LABEL'S REPUTATION FOR PURE LUXURY PRECEDES THEM.

1

2

1 Tan leather briefcase. 2 Constance mini in alligator.
3 Steve bag. 4 Brown crocodile Birkin bag. 5 Yohji38
in tan barenia calfskin. 6 Lindy30 handbag in graphite
crocodile.

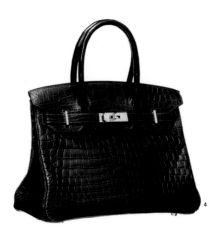

4

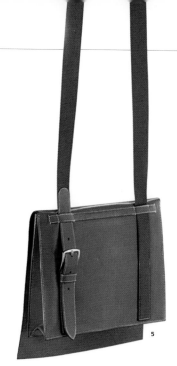

5

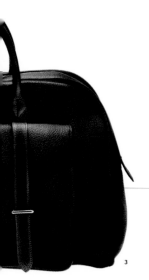

3

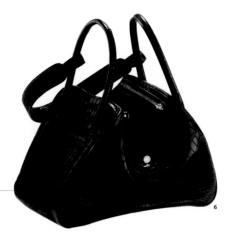

6

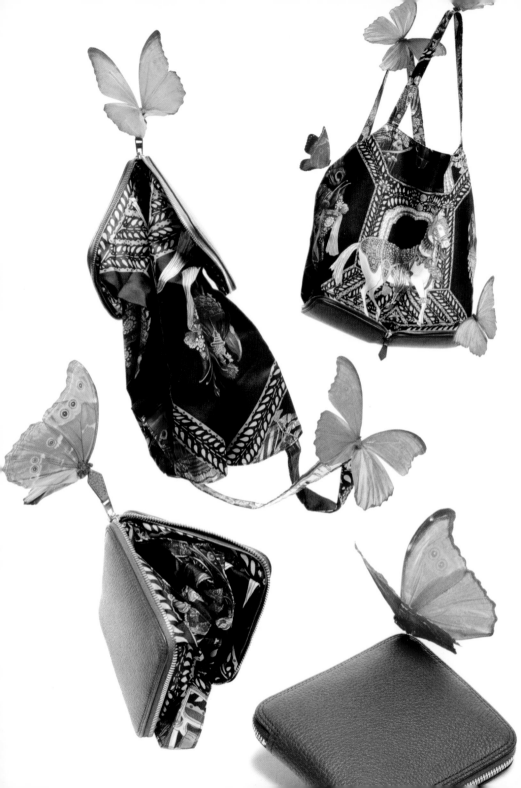

Hermès creates some of the most exquisitely crafted handbags in the world, and is responsible for two of the most iconic bags of all time, among the first to bear instantly recognizable and memorable names, the Kelly and the Birkin.

Founded in 1837 by Thierry Hermès, the Hermès company began life by making fine leather goods such as saddles and harnesses for the equestrian market. However, in keeping with the shift in modes of transport that occurred at the turn of the century, Monsieur Hermès began creating luggage, trunks and bags for the motoring industry. It was this shift of focus that eventually led to the creation of the first Hermès handbag in 1922.

Instantly recognizable by its logo depicting a Duc carriage with horse, the prestigious nature of an Hermès handbag derives from reputation, price and workmanship. The house's dedication to quality and luxury are the result of two guiding principles. First, Hermès has been a family-run enterprise since its inception, allowing it to maintain its focus on good craftsmanship. Secondly, the company does not employ assembly lines. All luggage and handbag collections are handmade, and typically a craftsman will only work on one handbag at a time.

Emphasis on quality craftsmanship, use of rare materials and the intensive nature of the production line means that it can take between 18 and 24 hours of skilled labour to create one Hermès handbag. The leathers employed by Hermès, ranging from alligator and lizard to buffalo and deer, are treated at the company's storage facility in Paris, France, where up to 600,000 skins are kept in a rigorously controlled environment. Hermès' design office is also constantly researching new materials and techniques for producing different finishes and effects.

Hermès has maintained its reputation as a pure luxury brand through quality and exclusivity. This is further enhanced by the Hermès distribution model, which ensures that its bags are only available through its own boutiques and not through franchises or independent retailers.

Hermès is comprised of 14 product divisions, which include scarves, ties, fragrances, menswear, womenswear and tableware. However, its most famous, recognizable and desirable items are the Birkin and Kelly handbags, named after Jane Birkin and Grace Kelly respectively. The Birkin bag is the result of the 1984 collaboration between Hermès and Jane Birkin, the British-born actress and singer and resident of France who complained that she could not find a bag to suit her. Instantly recognizable for its large, supple carryall shape, it is equally renowned for its use of precious metals such as gold or palladium for hardware, which, unlike silver, do not tarnish.

The Birkin bag's older cousin, the Kelly bag, is arguably the world's most coveted bag. Renamed the Kelly in 1956, after Grace Kelly used her large-model Hermès crocodile bag to hide her pregnancy from the press, it is seen, like many Hermès bags, to be one of the few designer handbags to maintain its value. Original 1956 productions of the Kelly bag consistently sell for around £4,000 (US $6,000) at auction. The Kelly now has a family tree that extends through eight sizes, from the original Kelly at 50 cm (20 in) to the Mini Kelly at 15 cm (6 in).

For its Autumn/Winter 08/9 collection, Hermès launched the Yohji bag in collaboration with designer Yohji Yamamoto. Designed as a messenger bag in smooth calfskin, the Yohji combines the modern design aesthetic of Yamamoto with the historical techniques of Hermès. In keeping with the pure luxury and exclusivity of Hermès, the Yohji bag has been produced as a limited edition and made available only through four Hermès boutiques in Paris, Tokyo, New York and London.

Desired by so many yet obtainable by so few, an Hermès handbag transcends the tastes of different generations and different countries. In an industry that is expected to respond to the demand for designs with mass appeal, Hermès understands that the fundamentals of matchless craftsmanship and refined elegance will never lose their attraction.

OPPOSITE SilkyPop bag. The calfskin wallet opens out to form a silk carryall.

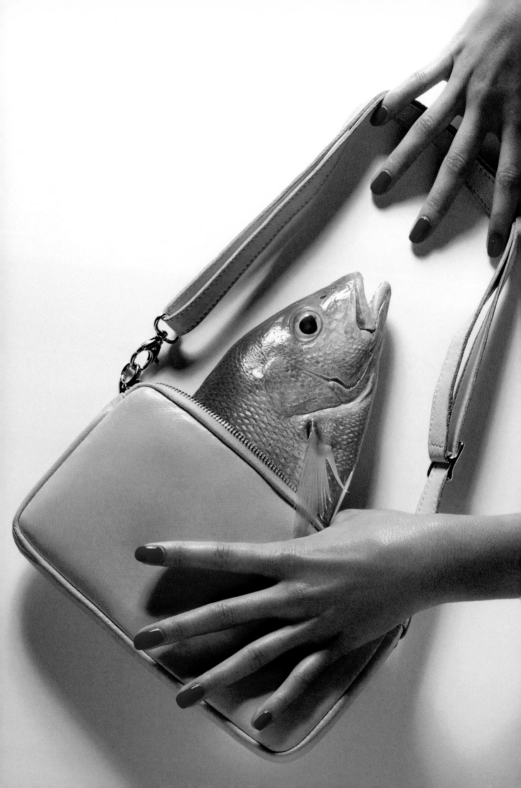

ISAAC REINA

With his fascination for the industrial world
and a strong attraction to accessories
design, Isaac Reina creates bags that
combine a rigorous technical approach
with playful wit.

OPPOSITE #035, S/S 08.

Founded in 2006
www.isaacreina.com

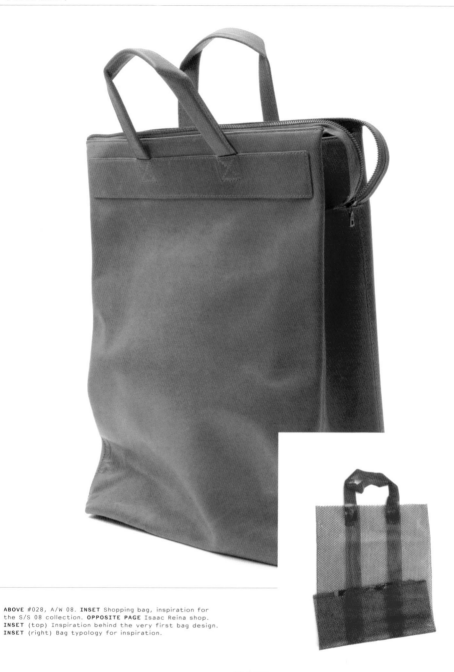

ABOVE #028, A/W 08. **INSET** Shopping bag, inspiration for
the S/S 08 collection. **OPPOSITE PAGE** Isaac Reina shop.
INSET (top) Inspiration behind the very first bag design.
INSET (right) Bag typology for inspiration.

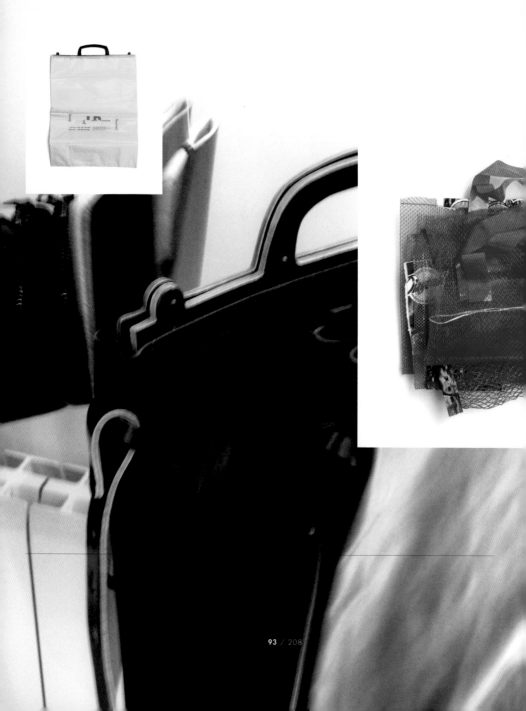

BY COMBINING THE INDUSTRIAL AESTHETIC OF BASIC PACKAGING WITH THE TRADITIONAL TECHNIQUES OF A LEATHER MASTER CRAFTSMAN, REINA SUCCEEDS IN CREATING THE EPITOME OF UNDERSTATED LUXURY.

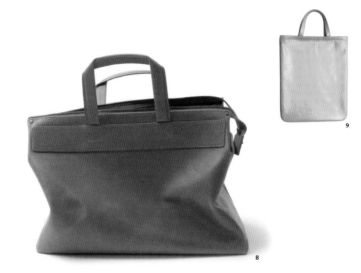

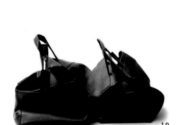

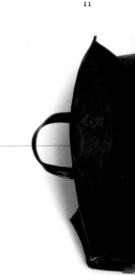

1 #068, A/W 08/09. 2 #028, S/S 08. 3 #011, A/W 07/08.
4 #028 and #110, A/W 08/09. 5 #028, A/W 06/07. 6 #014,
S/S 07. 7 #014, S/S 07. 8 #043, A/W 08/09. 9 #068, S/S
08. 10 #014 and 043, A/W 08/09. 11 #110, A/W 08/09.
12 #014, A/W 06/07.

Spanish-born Isaac Reina's purist style combines the three fundamental rules of good design – shape, proportion and material – with the skills he honed during his seven years at French luxury brand Hermès.

How long have you been designing?

'I have been designing bags since 2006.'

How did you initially get into bag design?

'Although I started out as a clothing designer, I have always been very attracted to and interested in fashion accessories. Bag design is quite similar to industrial or furniture design, and this is a way of working which seems to suit me — it's a good balance between fashion fantasy and serious industry.'

Do you have a certain process when working on your collections?

'My particular process is to keep working at something. I like considering and reviewing my last designs in order to evolve and improve them.'

Describe your techniques.

'When designing I utilize traditional techniques. I get very excited when researching old and new manufacturing techniques for bags and products in general. It's a real passion for me to learn. I always keep my eyes open in order to be inspired by the simplest or most sophisticated things — not just fashion of course, but contemporary art, architecture and design in general. I like combining a rigorous technical approach with a more playful, free contemporary one.'

What is your signature design style?

'The simpler the style, the better. Functionality is also important, however proportions can sometimes prove to be a bit of a challenge — too big, too slim, too small. I tend to keep detailing to a minimum while the quality has to be the best possible.'

What inspires you and where do you find your inspiration?

'I find myself inspired by many things at once. These include everyday objects that are too often taken for granted, such as mass industrial design.

I like looking at vintage bags that I find in flea markets because they represent manufacturing techniques considered to be too complicated to use in this day and age, and also the works of industrial designers from the 1960s and 1970s.'

What materials/fabrications do you use?

'I use basic leathers such as simple classic calfskin, a pure material for creating shape, pattern and proportion.'

What are your plans and ambitions for the future?

'I plan to continue designing bags. I consider myself to be very lucky because I'm a young brand, creating quality bags that I find really interesting. Of course I do have other ambitions, for example to expand my existing collection with the introduction of a footwear line.'

How do you feel about the bag industry and how do you think it is going to develop in the future?

'The bag industry is booming at the moment, with big name brands spending thousands to push their products into magazines and window displays. I want my approach to be the exact opposite, and maintain my business on a small, intimate scale.'

Do you have any thoughts on the so-called IT bag? For example, has it run its course? Is there still room for it in the market?

'IT bags seem to be designed as a marketing tool. They can often be aesthetically pleasing and introduce new ideas or proportions, however a lot seem to be overshadowed by publicity, regardless of their quality — it's such a shame. There is no denying, however, that the IT bag has become a kind of flagship for all brands.'

OPPOSITE #059, S/S 08.

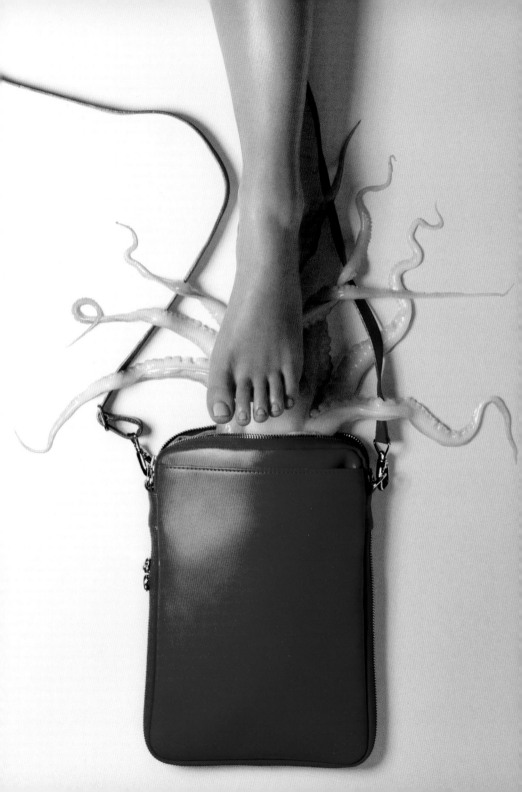

JAMIN PUECH

French label Jamin Puech is the perfect
antidote to a market that is fast becoming
homogenized. Its unique look is a result of
the techniques created by the label's
worldwide network of craftsmen.

CLOCKWISE FROM TOP LEFT Akil, S/S 09; Abakoum,
A/W 08/09; Azah, S/S 09.

Founded in 1990
www.jamin-puech.com

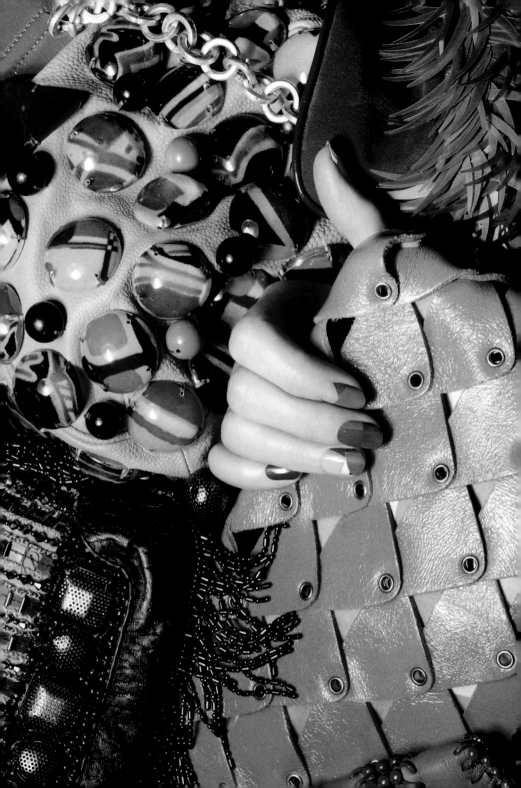

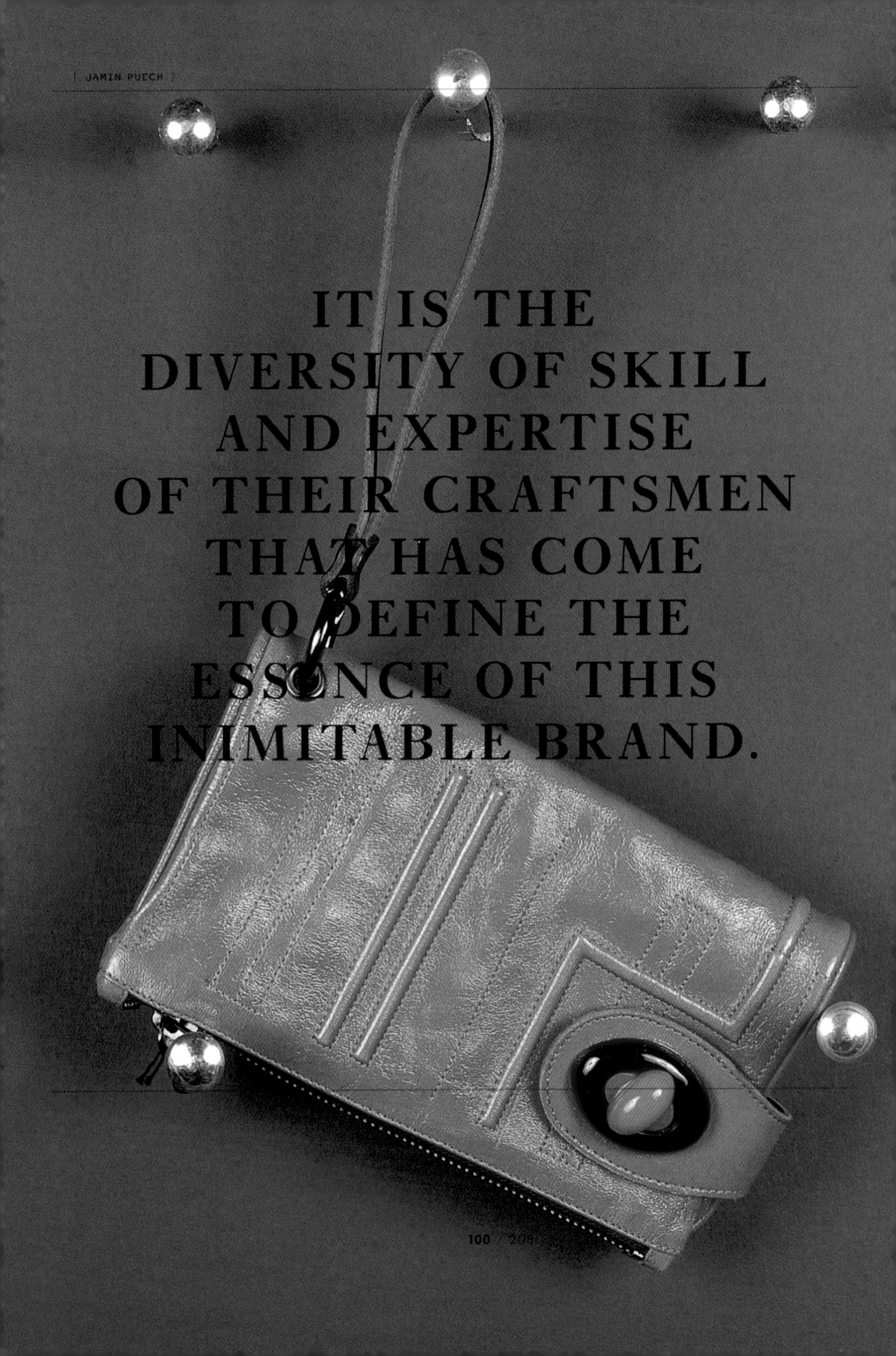

IT IS THE
DIVERSITY OF SKILL
AND EXPERTISE
OF THEIR CRAFTSMEN
THAT HAS COME
TO DEFINE THE
ESSENCE OF THIS
INIMITABLE BRAND.

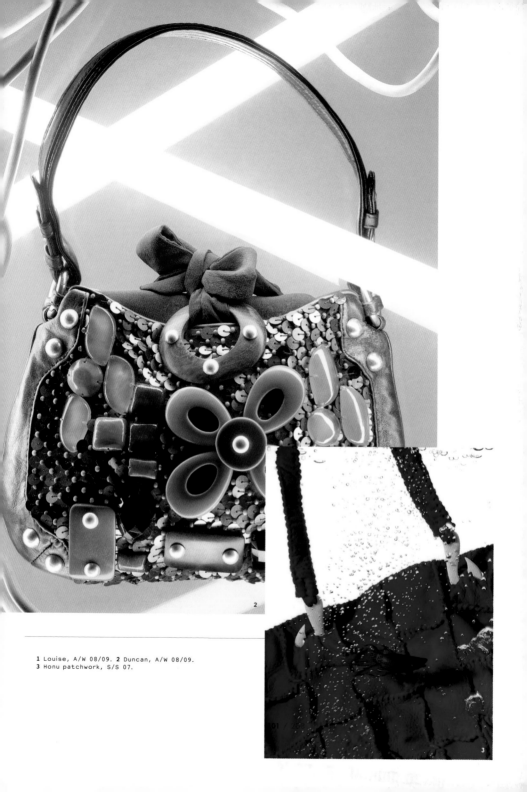

1 Louise, A/W 08/09. **2** Duncan, A/W 08/09.
3 Honu patchwork, S/S 07.

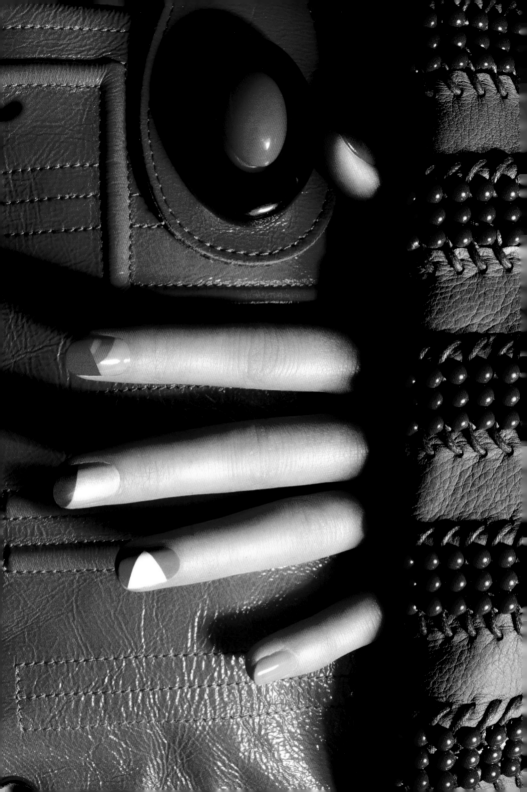

Established in 1990 by French design duo Benoît Jamin and Isabelle Puech, this eponymous label successfully mixes mainstream western style with influences from other cultures.

How long have you been designing for, and when did you start you own business?

'Jamin Puech was created in 1990 in Paris. We started to design and make bags and jewellery a few months before, for the Balmain fashion show. In 1991, we showed our first collection at the Salon Premiere Classe exhibition thanks to the Festival of Young Creators in Hyeres, where we won first prize. In 1996 we opened our first boutique in Paris.'

Do you have a certain process for working on the collections? For example, do you sketch first or make models of the bags?

'We start by drawing, then work on the patterns and create the shape to see how the fabric or leather reacts to it. We then work with the prototype, making any changes necessary until everything is exactly as we want it.'

Describe the Jamin Puech signature style.

'Our bags are faithful to the Parisian tradition and are inspired by 21st century fashion designers such as Paul Poiret, Elsa Schiaparelli, Yves Saint Laurent and Jean Paul Gaultier. Our signature style has to be whimsical, witty and humorous. The recipe for our French style is savoir vivre, allure, elegance, nonchalance and spontaneity — after all they are only bags, it's not art. You have to have fun with it.'

What inspires you, and where do you find your inspiration?

'Our inspiration comes from everything: exhibitions, movies, books that we read, interesting people, travel. We have small antennas on our heads and catch whatever is interesting.'

Do you have any designer favourites or heroes?

'There are quite a few designers we like for their style, personality and approach to fashion: Martin Margiela, Alexander McQueen, Dries Van Noten, John Galliano and many more.'

What materials and fabrications do you use?

'Our bags combine traditional and modern materials such as raffia, rattan, macramé, wood, nacre, horn and plastic. Leather has come back into fashion thanks to new and modern treatments such as stretch, moulded, tattooed or thermo-changing leathers. Reptile skins and furs complete our ongoing quest for new materials. This mix of materials and textures give our collections a really unique style.'

Are you planning to expand your business by introducing new lines and collections?

'This year we opened three new shops in London, Barcelona and Osaka respectively. We always have a few bags for men in the collection. These have proved to be particularly popular with our Japanese clients. Every season, we introduce a new range of products — luggage, clothing, accessories, shoes, scarves or jewellery — it just depends on our mood!'

How do you feel about the bag industry at the moment? Will customers be looking for a quick fix or something with longevity?

'The most important thing for us is the "coup de foudre" (love at first sight) and relationship between the client and the bag. Clients visit our stores to find an exclusive bag they will fall in love with. They are looking for a bag they won't find on every woman in the street and one that will make them feel special, knowing that they are wearing an original creation.'

Do you have any thoughts on the so-called IT bag? Has it run its course or is there still room for an IT bag?

'We never follow trends or make IT bags. Clients buy our bags because they like them, some of them become IT bags because of the quantity ordered or sold, but it is the client who determines our "it" and not us — we let them decide.'

OPPOSITE (left) Louise, A/W 08/09; (right) Kameron, S/S 09.

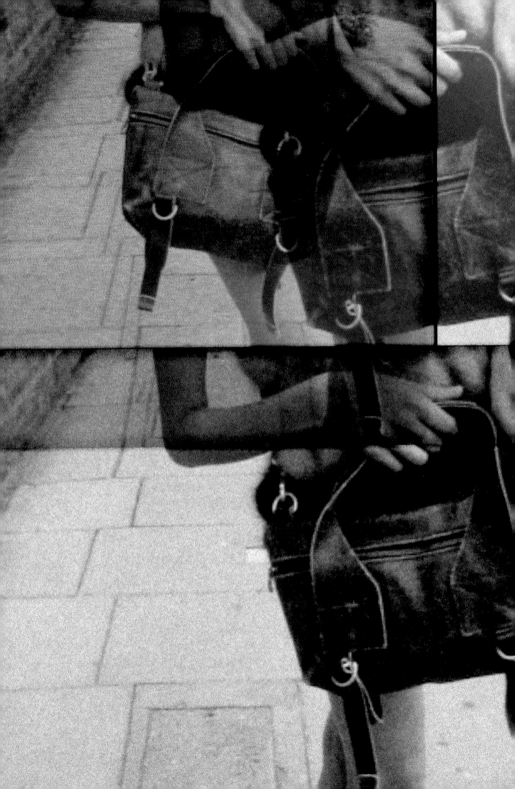

Jas M.B. bags are stylish without trying to be. As one of the UK's leading and most accomplished bag designers, founder Jas Sehmbi points to practicality and simplicity as the qualities most central to his design.

JAS M.B.

OPPOSITE Old School messenger bags.

Founded in 2000
www.doorsbyjasmb.com

BUILT TO LAST AND DESIGNED TO MANAGE WOMEN'S EVERYDAY LIVES, JAS M.B. BAGS ARE EFFORTLESSLY STYLISH AND TIMELESS.

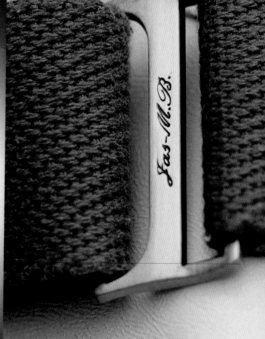

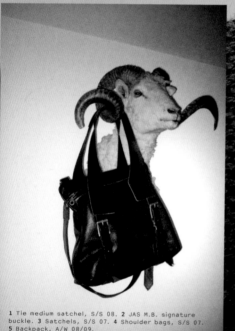

1 Tie medium satchel, S/S 08. 2 JAS M.B. signature buckle. 3 Satchels, S/S 07. 4 Shoulder bags, S/S 07. 5 Backpack, A/W 08/09.

1

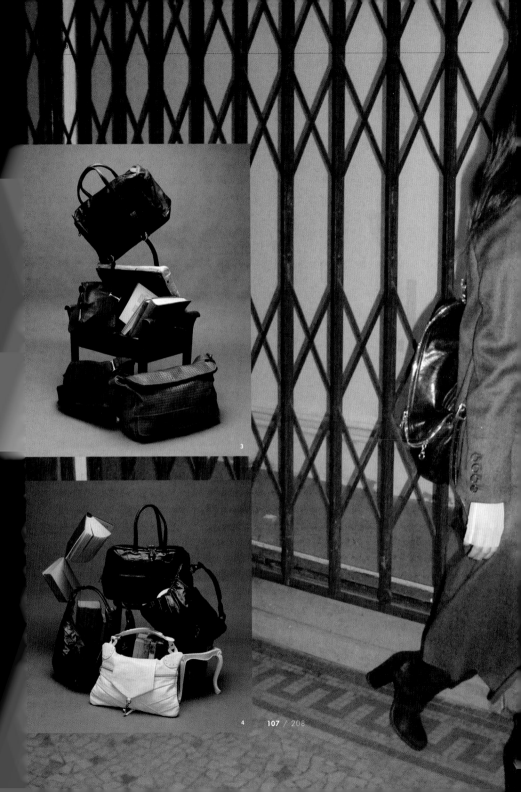

African-born Jas Sehmbi moved to India as a child before settling in the UK in 1970. Three months after graduating from an art foundation course in East London Jas was retailing small leather and canvas bags, and in 1995 he opened his first store. In 1993 Sehmbi established himself as a leading accessories designer when he created the first ever DJ bag. Initially working in nylon and canvas, by the time he launched the Jas M.B. brand in 2000 he was working solely with fine Italian leather and was becoming known for the weightless construction of his bags.

'I wanted to see guys carrying bags in the UK',

Sehmbi says of the launch of his initial male-only line. This unique approach to the market underpins the philosophy of the Jas M.B. brand, which is about creating opportunities and opening doors. The designer now prefers to think of his bags as unisex, although he does design a few exclusively feminine pieces for particular clients and stores such as New York's famous Barneys.

Versatility is an important consideration in Sehmbi's designs, and colour is no exception.

'We always try to keep our colours as subtle as possible',

he explains,

'because that way they can be worn at any time of the day'.

If designing especially for men, Sehmbi applies a particularly understated colour palette:

'As far as men's bags go, I feel that they are still not fully accepting of more adventurous colours, and shapes and constructions still have to remain soft and functional. Men are always looking for things that are practical, much more than women.'

Sehmbi's major source of inspiration is the Industrial Revolution, a time when production and manufacturing were driven by this sense of practicality and need. The designer's desire for his bags to be highly function-driven is also evident in his attitude to hardware:

'I used to design a lot of hardware but I've recently cut down. I feel the simpler and lighter the bag, the more useful it will be.'

The brand's signature style bowling bag is as popular today as it was when it was first launched, a testament to the designer's ability to create designs with longevity and wearability as well as practicality.

Sehmbi will often carry styles over from previous seasons, offering them in fresh new colours and finishes rather than feeling the need to introduce new styles every season.

'I will look at a piece of technical engineering or a piece of aggressive looking jewellery and think about how I would transform it, making it softer and more malleable to the touch.'

This tactile approach naturally influences his design process:

'The most important thing is the feel and then the look and texture of the leather',

explains Sehmbi,

'for me the feel of the leather is even more important than the colour'.

In 2003 the Doors by Jas M.B. boutique opened in the heart of London's Soho. The aptly named store represents the doors Sehmbi has opened (and continues to open) for graduates wanting to work in the fashion industry. In keeping with the philosophy of his store, Sehmbi is also keen on collaborative projects. These include an exclusive range of eco-friendly bags developed with designer Katharine Hamnett. Manufactured with chrome-free leather, organic cotton lining and nickel-free brass hardware, the collaborative line's key styles include the Adi and Pyramid bags.

The brand more recently launched a limited edition range called 'Love Jas', which was initially only available at Topshop's flagship store on London's Oxford Street. Offering the same outstanding qualities as the Jas M.B. main line but at a more affordable price range, 'Love Jas' is another sign of the brand's versatility.

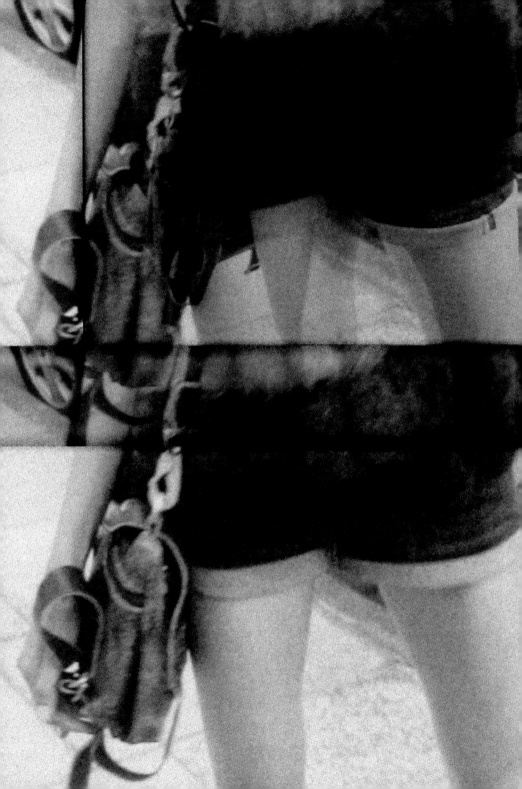

JÉRÔME DREYFUSS

Slouchy, relaxed shapes with minimal
hardware focus on function and practicality
and are quietly luxurious — letting the bag
design and beautifully soft leather do
the talking.

OPPOSITE Tom in lambskin, A/W 08/09.

Founded in 2002
www.jerome-dreyfuss.com

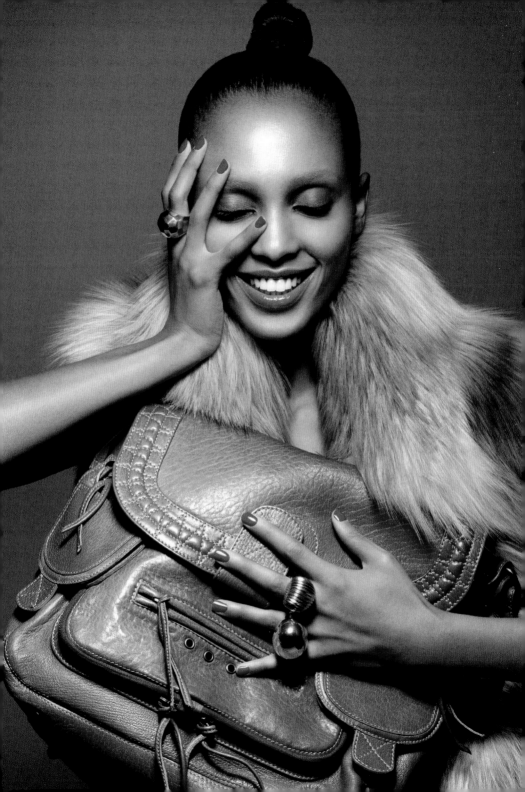

'I DO WHAT I FEEL. I'M TRYING TO HELP WOMEN ORGANIZE THEIR LIVES'

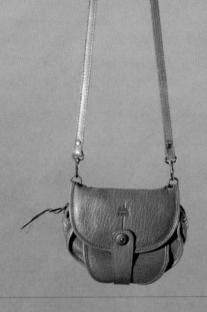

1 MOMO in fire lambskin, S/S 09. 2 Bernard in fire
lambskin, S/S 08. 3 Andre in pebble karung skin, S/S 07.
4 Franky in khaki lambskin, A/W 08/09. 5 Selection from
S/S 08 collection.

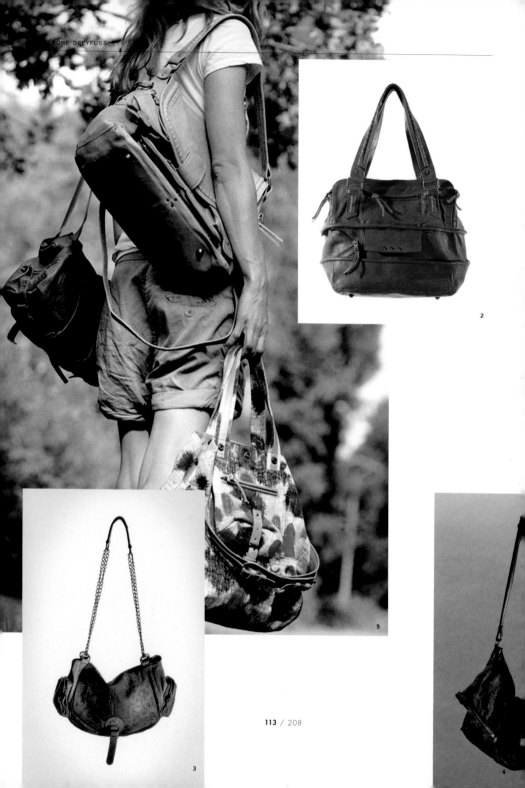

2

5

3

4

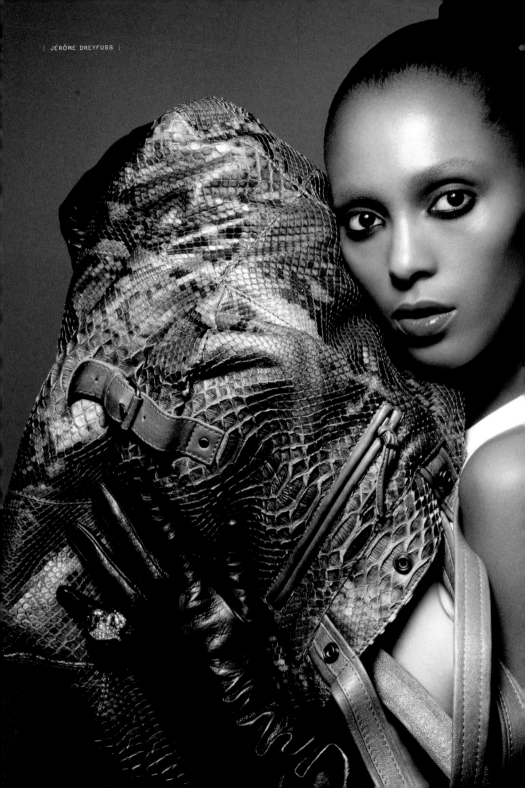

A fashion designer turned accessories designer, Jérôme Dreyfuss launched his self-titled bag label in 2002, and quickly established himself as the antidote to the overly branded and fussy bags that were popular at the time.

At the heart of the Jérôme Dreyfuss brand is the designer's commitment to ecologically produced leathers. In 2006 he launched the Agricouture label, which champions production techniques that respect the environment. From responsibly breeding animals for leather to producing the finished product, Jérôme Dreyfuss promotes the preservation of nature and healthy manufacturing conditions.

How long have you been designing for?

'I began designing when I was around 12 years old. I started creating dresses in 1988 and designing bags in 2002.'

How did you get into bag design?

'I worked for John Galliano for a year as one of his assistants and then worked for the Elite Model Agency in Paris for two years. I got into bag design by watching my girlfriends and wife, who were not interested in structured, heavy, logo-type bags'.

Do you have a certain process when working on your collections? Do you sketch first or make models of the bags?

'I make sketches, play with the leather, the colours, everything at the same time. I run my company during the day and I work on my bags at the end of the day and night. I enjoy the whole process — I just love doing my job.'

Describe your techniques. For example, what type of constructions do you use, what's the inspiration?

'I structure my bags in the way that I learned to structure dresses. I want the construction to be as fluid as dresses, as well as highly practical.'

What is your signature design style?

'Softness, lightness, practicality, always with three or four little rivets on the intersection of the double top-stitching. I only use really soft ecological lambskins with a lot of colours. Billy, the first bag I designed, is still my bestseller. It is made of leather that is as soft as a baby's skin. My bags are known for their softness and lightness'.

What inspires you and where do you find your inspiration?

'My wife, my friends, Africa, architecture and furniture designers such as Jean Prouvé, Charlotte Perriand, Nogushi, Georges Nelson from the 1960s; my house on the river in the countryside; designers such as Thierry Mugler, Azzedine Alaia, Claude Montana ... Why? Because they made me dream when I was 15.'

What materials and fabrics do you use? Do you have a signature leather you always use in your collections?

'Vegetal lambskin. I only use ecological lambskins. I'm trying to use only clean and vegetal products to tan the skins. I LOVE MY PLANET! I use one piece of leather to make each bag, with minimal hardware. Function rather than decoration makes the aesthetic.'

What are your plans and ambitions for the future?

'After the opening of my first store in Paris, I'm thinking of opening new ones in Paris and New York. And maybe a little clothing line again.'

How do you feel about the bag industry at the moment and how do you think it is going to develop? Will customers be looking for a quick fix or something with longevity?

'I feel bags are what perfumes used to be in the 1980s. But I think there is still a long way to go with bags. Luxury equals longevity, but fashion and style change every six months.'

Do you have any thoughts on the so called IT bag? How would you define an IT bag?

'It has to be worn by Paris Hilton! I don't care for IT bags and I'm happy not to be known for them.'

How would you define luxury?

Luxury is artisanal, rareness, a dream.

OPPOSITE Large Billy bag in python skin, A/W 08/09.

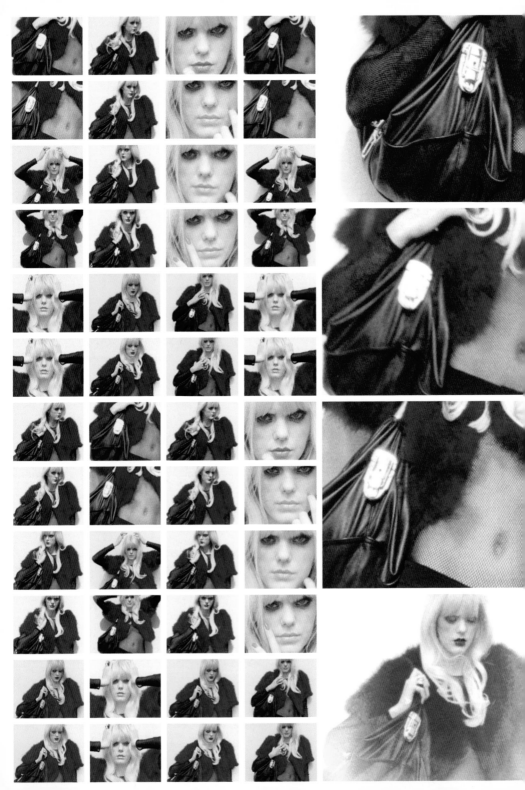

This avant garde German design house is synonymous with beautifully constructed, modern and stylish bags that unite German utilitarianism and French luxury.

KAVIAR GAUCHE

OPPOSITE Square bag, A/W 08/09.

Founded in 2004
www.kaviargauche.com

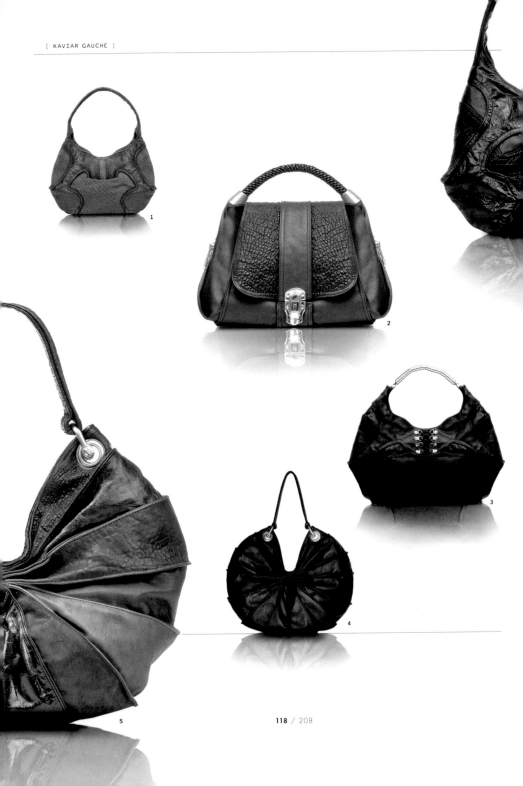

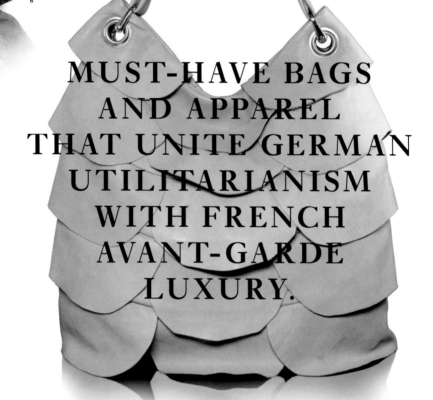

6

MUST-HAVE BAGS AND APPAREL THAT UNITE GERMAN UTILITARIANISM WITH FRENCH AVANT-GARDE LUXURY.

7

1 Broiler bag, 'casual', A/W 08/09. 2 Square bag,
A/W 08/09. 3 Broiler bag, A/W 08/09. 4 Lamella bag,
classic style launched 2004. 5 Lamella bag, 'mixed',
A/W 08/09. 6 Broiler bag, 'burgundy', A/W 08/09.
7 Scale bag, S/S 09.

Founded in 2004 by Berlin-based Alexandra Fischer-Roehler and Johanna Kühl, and currently enjoying international acclaim, Kaviar Gauche has become one of Germany's most notable and successful young brands.

Having graduating from the Esmod Fashion School in Berlin, Fischer-Roehler and Kühl initially went their separate ways, honing their individual skills in the fashion world. Fischer-Roehler's graduation collection was honoured at the Moët & Chandon Fashion Awards in 2003, while Kühl began work in London for Vivienne Westwood before moving to Paris to assist Martine Sitbon. It was in 2004 that the duo teamed up to form the Kaviar Gauche label.

Fischer-Roehler and Kühl describe their aesthetic as a

'connection between luxury and the avant-garde'

– a description that also informs their choice of name. Derived from the name of French jet-setting society, *gauche caviar*, 'Kaviar Gauche' is drawn from an expression used in France to refer to 'champagne socialists'.

Revolutionary design ideals set the scene for the duo's first collection; a guerrilla-style fashion show in front of the popular Parisian department store Colette. They rented a flat near the chic boutique, hung loudspeakers out of the windows and presented their debut collection. A huge success, the show attracted a great deal of press and publicity and – most importantly – secured their first order with New York's prestigious department store Barneys.

Although they initially studied apparel design, the duo find a greater sense of flexibility and spontaneity in designing accessories.

'Designing handbags means more freedom for innovative forms',

they explain. Inspired by contrary themes from their everyday surroundings, in particular by nature, the designers' strong affinity for bold organic forms is instantly recognizable in their dynamic bag constructions and strong material choices.

With minimal hardware and no obvious branding, a Kaviar Gauche bag speaks for itself. Statuesque silhouettes are combined with intricately designed construction work inspired by the designers' fascination with organic forms. Contrasts also play a big part in the duo's design process, particularly in their choice of materials. Combining highly textured leather with super smooth surfaces and matt with semi-shine leathers highlights the skilfully designed pattern cutting, while the use of subtle tones of similar colours adds further depth to the designs. Although the focus is on construction, the pair do employ touches of decoration with studs and Swarovski crystals, either used all over or as block placement.

Kaviar Gauche focuses on the relationship between bags and apparel, adopting a new perspective on the traditional convention of matching a bag with an outfit. The designers connect apparel and bags by drawing attention to the intrinsic links between the two, adding bag elements to clothes and clothing characteristics to bags. The signature Lamella bag, for example, perfectly encapsulates the designers' style. Created by employing a technique that was originally intended to be used for a skirt, forming strips of different types of leather into a distinctive crescent shape, the Lamella successful marries aspects of apparel and accessory.

The designers count top model Nadja Auermann and German actress Heike Makatsch among their celebrity fans, and yet prefer to work without the influence of trend:

'we have worked independently from the first moment and we hope that we will continue to work in the same way.'

Having already won recognition with a number of international awards, and selling successfully in more than ten cities across the globe, Fischer-Roehler and Kühl have big plans for the future. These include a diffusion line for their younger customers, an expansion of their apparel line, and expanding their accessory line into footwear.

OPPOSITE (left) Swarovski Lamella bag, S/S 08; (right) Lamella bag classic, 2004; (below) Laughing Face bag, S/S 07.

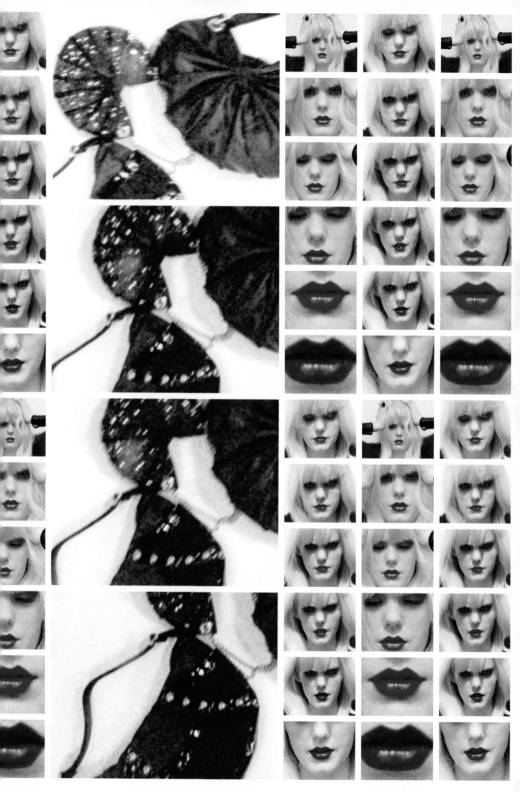

LARA BOHINC

Lara Bohinc made her name with her architectural jewellery designs before expanding into the luxury bag market. Drawing inspiration from her jewellery, her signature bags are distinctive in their use of decorative hardware and intricate craftmanship.

OPPOSITE Solar Eclipse in ivory, S/S 09.

Founded in 1997
www.larabohinc107.co.uk

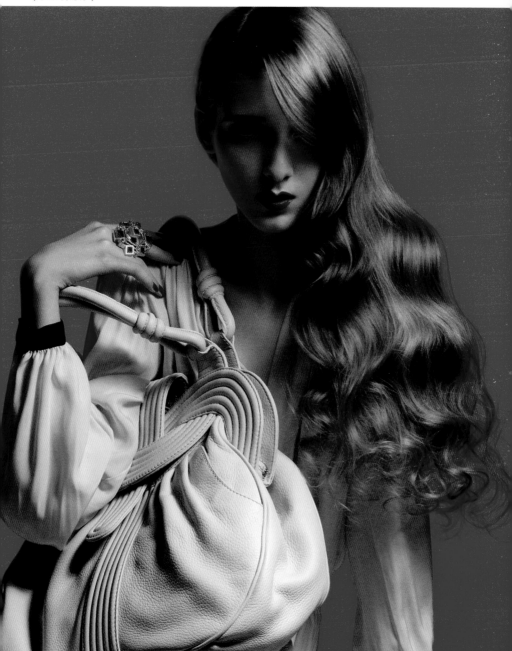

HER DESIGNS ARE MODERN AND TIMELESS, EDGY YET BEAUTIFUL, EMBELLISHED BUT WITH CLEAN LINES, AND ALWAYS FEATURING THE HIGHEST QUALITY MATERIALS AND EXPERT CRAFTSMANSHIP.

1 Lunar Eclipse in ivory deer leather, S/S 08–S/S 09.
2 Apollo tote in smoke patent leather, A/W 08/09.
3 Nadia in ivory deer leather, S/S 08–S/S 09.
4 Solar Eclipse in black printed ostrich leather, S/S 09.
5 Laretta bag in metallic silver calf leather, A/W 07/08–
S/S 09. 6 Solar Eclipse in gold python, S/S 09–A/W 09/10.

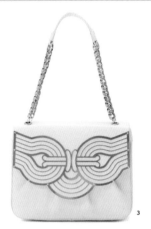

3

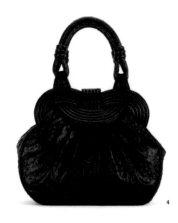

4

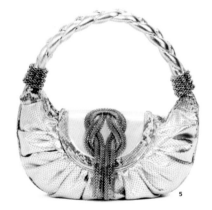

5

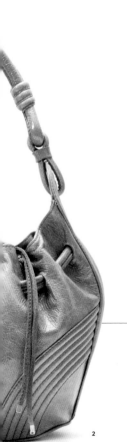

2

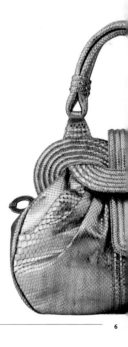

6

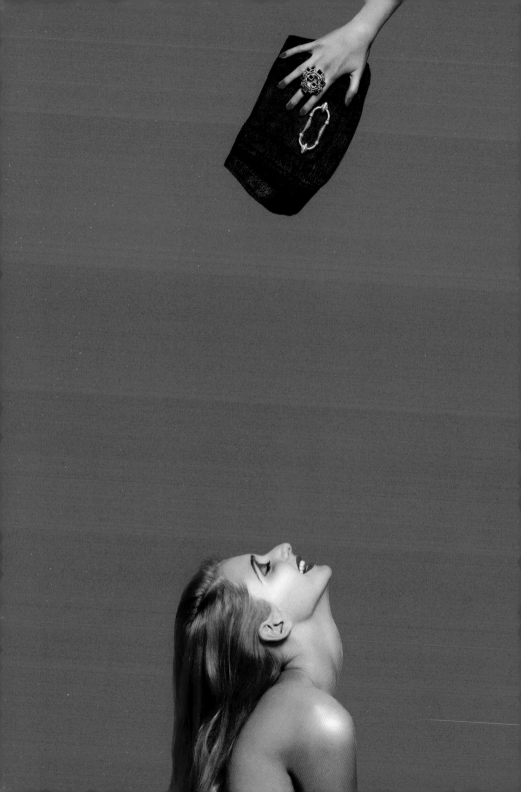

Born in Slovenia in 1972, Lara Bohinc studied industrial design at the Academy for Arts in Ljubljana, followed by an MA in jewellery and metal work at the Royal Academy of Arts in London. She debuted her jewellery collection at London Fashion Week in 1997 and quickly established herself as a leading cutting-edge jewellery designer. She has collaborated with numerous fashion luminaries over the years including Gucci, Lanvin and Guy Laroche, as well as acting as a consultant for Cartier, while her designs are worn by high-profile celebrities from Madonna and Sarah Jessica Parker to the more avant garde Roisin Murphy and Bjork.

Bohinc is something of an anomaly in the world of luxury bags. Her designs are modern and timeless, edgy yet beautiful, embellished but with clean lines, and always featuring the highest quality materials and expert craftmanship. Although considered a young brand at just over ten years old, she has established herself as one of the most exciting European brands within the luxury goods sector with her growing range of jewellery, leather accessories, bags and sunglasses.

Bohinc debuted her bag range in 2005, naturally drawing on her jewellery work for inspiration. The brand is best known for its signature Lunar Eclipse bag, which is directly drawn from the Lunar Eclipse jewellery range, with the lines of the chains translated into leather profiles on the bags.

Bohinc created an exclusive python collection of the Eclipse to be sold only at Harvey Nichols, which was the first exclusive Lara Bohinc collection to be launched. The loops and twists synonymous with the Eclipse jewellery collection were translated onto the bags, and the only metal component featured is a custom designed brass zip fixture that takes its inspiration from the Eclipse Apollo pendant.

The Laratella bag is also directly inspired by the jewellery range – the Laratella bracelet from the brand's Marina collection. Using jewellery instead of pre-made hardware on the bags makes Bohinc's work truly unique.

Bohinc explains that

'Hardware is important to the look of the brand, but is more about decoration than function. In our Laratella bag it was all about the hardware. In the Lunar range the hardware was translated into leather.'

Depending on the collection, Bohinc utilizes both soft and hard constructions. While her use of materials varies, embracing calf leather, lambskin, deerskin, python and ostrich, snakeskin is a perennial favourite.

'I use one leather per bag otherwise it proves to be a logistical nightmare at the production stage,' she says.

'But I do prefer to use more than one leather.'

Bohinc's Autumn/Winter 09/10 collection was inspired by bubbles and clouds, which translated into a bubble tote with laser-cut layers of clouds in goat leather with brass buckles. For Spring/Summer 09 she produced the Tatum, an Art Deco style design in calf leather with a croco print in soft grey and white, embellished with a satin gold-plated buckle.

Discussing the trend for IT bags, Bohinc believes

'that era is over, people are looking for something more discrete now. Customers are now looking for something with longevity, classic styles that will last'.

Bohinc believes that the definition of true luxury is

'items that make you feel special and unique because of the high attention to detail, quality of manufacture, top of the range materials and uniqueness of design. Something that isn't a necessity in life but something that makes life look, taste and feel better.'

Lara Bohinc's strikingly beautiful designs definitely make life look better.

OPPOSITE Tatum clutch in charcoal grey, S/S 09.

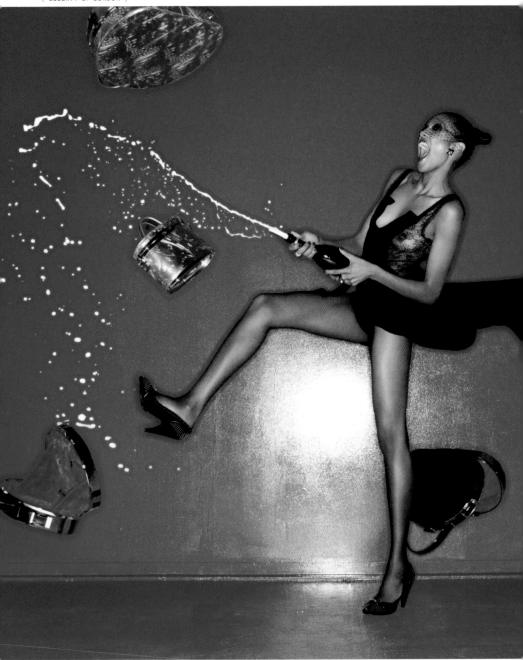

LIBERTY OF LONDON

Utilizing materials such as fine soft leathers, and exotic python and alligator for the limited-edition bags, each collection is unique without losing any of the darkly romantic appeal associated with the heritage of the Liberty brand.

OPPOSITE (top to bottom) Turquoise lacquer embossed hat box bag; pink lacquer embossed vanity case; purple croc hat box; black croc leather oval box bag.

Founded in 2005
www.liberty.co.uk

CREATING BAGS THAT ARE MODERN AND DESIRABLE, LIBERTY OF LONDON DESIGNS RETAIN THE OPULENT AND EXOTIC SPIRIT OF THE LIBERTY NAME.

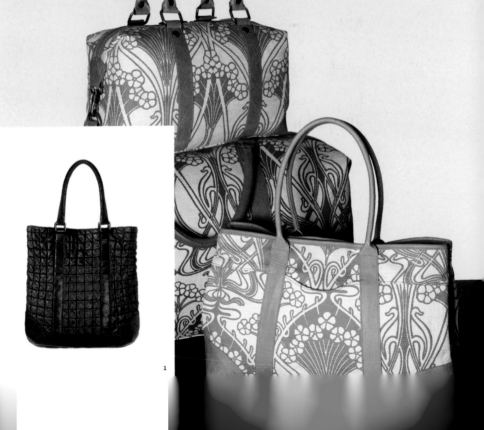

1

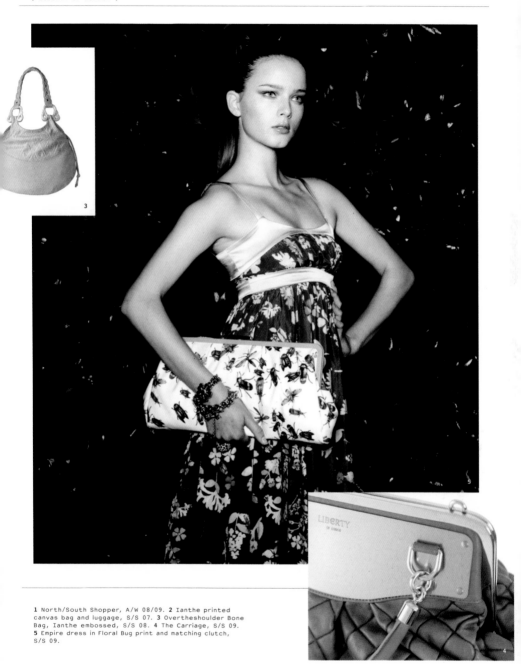

1 North/South Shopper, A/W 08/09. 2 Ianthe printed canvas bag and luggage, S/S 07. 3 Overtheshoulder Bone Bag, Ianthe embossed, S/S 08. 4 The Carriage, S/S 09. 5 Empire dress in Floral Bug print and matching clutch, S/S 09.

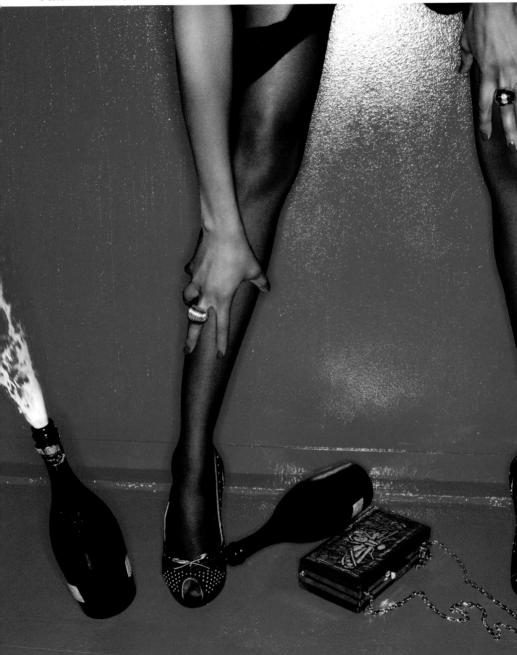

For a relatively new luxury accessories label, Liberty of London has a lot of history draw on. As the in-house label of renowned London department store Liberty, Liberty of London has a world-famous vintage print archive and artisanal heritage at its disposal.

One of London's oldest and most famous department stores, Liberty is a landmark in the British capital. Initially only selling ornaments, fabrics and art objects from Japan and the Far East, Liberty now stocks a mix of modern niche products. In September 2005 the store launched its first branded luxury accessory label, Liberty of London. Handbags and accessories are at the heart of the label, which also includes scarves, stationary, jewellery, swimwear, lingerie, menswear and a home collection. Developed by Creative Director Tamara Salman, the collection celebrates the store's history – in particular its experimentalism and love of all things from the East – from a modern point of view.

'I always start with the prints',

says Salman,

'I look back into the Liberty archives and take inspiration and reference from the oldest Liberty prints. It's then important to contemporize them and make them relevant for today.'

Archive Liberty prints are reconfigured and re-coloured and feature heavily in the new label's bag designs, bringing a new lease of life to some of the brand's most loved prints.

'The Art Nouveau Ianthe print is the signature print from Liberty of London',

says Salman.

'It comes through in every collection, but each season it is modified and updated to keep it fresh. I also ensure that the richness of the Liberty heritage comes through in embroidery, embossing and hardware.'

Known for its print and texture, the Liberty of London collection also explores new bag crafting techniques, which helps to ensure that the finish is both luxurious and unique. From digitally printing onto soft leather and embossing, to laser cutting and jewel embellishments, every bag is handcrafted with an individual style. Working closely with the best artisanal factories in Europe, the bags have a high level of workmanship, which is apparent from the exclusive woven and printed fabrics to the handcrafted metal work.

Each collection is comprised of a selection of bag styles, which are revisited each season in different colourways, fabrications and prints.

'The Box bag is our signature shape',

says Salman.

'These handmade structured bags portray a sense of glamour and decadence from the 1950s, however I always add in a twist and contemporary edge to make them relevant for today. I love using frames for bags – it is something quite hard to do beautifully and gives a real sense of hand craftsmanship. Liberty is about handcrafted beauty.'

Other bag styles include elegant clutches, shoppers and classic carriage bags such as an over-the-shoulder framed purse bag.

For such a young label, Liberty of London has come a long way in a short space of time. From its beginnings as the in-house label of one of the world's most famous department stores, the label is now stocked in over 150 boutiques and department stores worldwide. The brand's first stand-alone store on London's Sloane Street cements the label's status as a coveted and fast-growing luxury brand, fusing the artistic spirit of the original store with a modern bohemian style.

Salman speculates that in the past

'it was all about the IT bag and thankfully we never tried to create this look. Today the discerning customer is looking for something individual and unique in the luxury market. Customers want to buy a bag that will stand the test of time both in terms of its look and quality. I think people will be much more selective in the future. Instead of buying several bags, they will spend time looking for that single special purchase. I want bags that I have designed for Liberty of London to be pieces that are kept and cherished.'

OPPOSITE Floral Bugs Cigarette Clutch in purple and gold.

LOEWE

oewe is Spain's premium luxury brand.
Synonymous with quality, elegance and
sophistication, it is one of the oldest
luxury houses in the world.

OPPOSITE (Left to right) Ava in dark blue crocodile, A/W 08/09; Black velvet evening bag from Loewe archive, c.1910); Calle in pink ostrich, S/S 09.

Founded in 1846
www.loewe.com

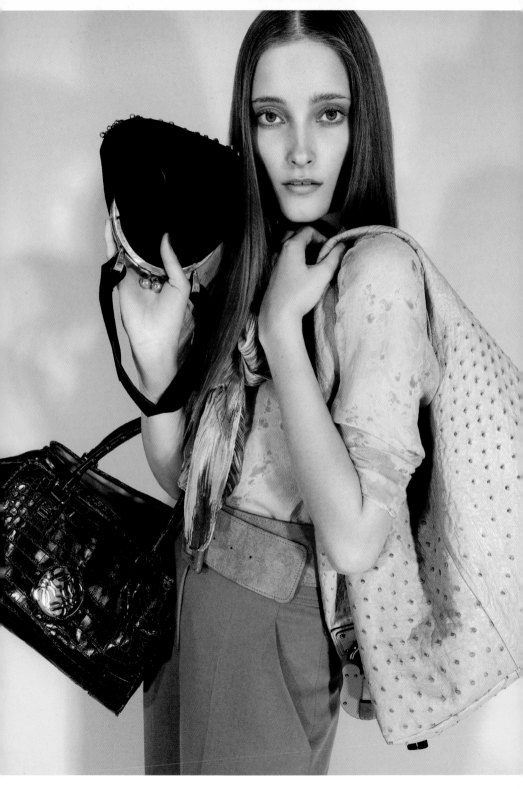

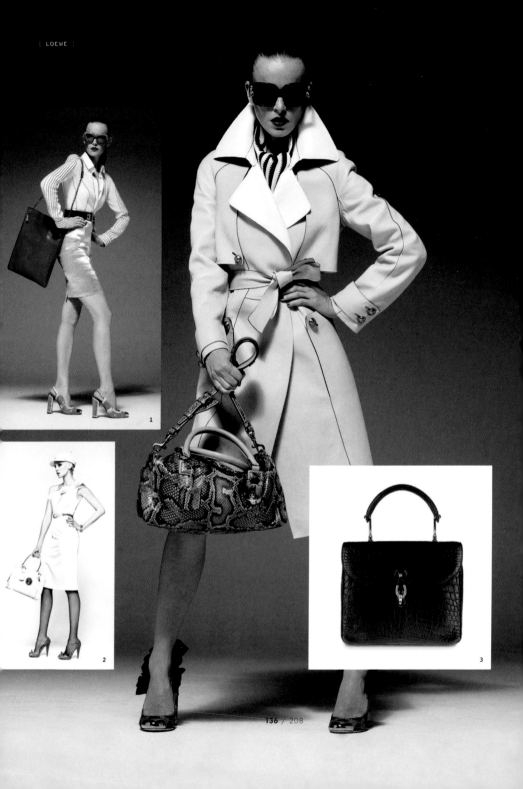

LOEWE IS SPAIN'S PREMIUM LUXURY BRAND, SYNONYMOUS WITH QUALITY, ELEGANCE AND SOPHISTICATION

1 Malt calfskin Paso bag, S/S 09. 2 White crocodile Ava bag, S/S 09. 3 Crocodile bag from the Loewe archives, c.1960 4 Python Ame bag, S/S 09. 5 Chalk Karung and Chain Gia 21 bag, S/S 09.

137 / 208

Predominantly a leather goods maker with a focus on artisanal craftsmanship, the Loewe label also boasts pret-a-porter lines for men and women, as well as footwear and accessories lines. Under the direction of design wunderkind Stuart Vevers, however, Loewe is entering a new chapter in its fascinating story.

In 1846 a group of artisans opened a workshop in Madrid and set about producing small leather goods such as men's purses, cigar holders and briefcases. It wasn't until almost 30 years later that the Loewe brand became fully established. When German leather designer Enrique Loewe Roessberg settled in Madrid, he became impressed by the knowledge and craftsmanship of these artisans and began working alongside them, fusing his method of work with their creative approach. Before long this collaboration gave birth to the Loewe label.

The first Loewe store was launched in Madrid in 1892, and quickly became known for its quality leather goods. Over the years Loewe became particularly renowned for its use of exotic leather skins such as snake, iguana and crocodile. In 1965 the label introduced a pret-a-porter line of clothing, designed by fashion luminaries Karl Lagerfeld (womenswear) and Giorgio Armani (menswear).

In 2008 Stuart Vevers became Creative Director at the luxury house. Vevers has worked for some of the world's most prestigious fashion brands, including Louis Vuitton, Bottega Venetta and Givenchy, but is perhaps most notable for transforming the fortunes of British luxury leather goods company Mulberry, turning it from an old-fashioned bag label into one of the most desirable accessories brands in the world.

Keen to establish an identity for Loewe while developing continuity within the brand's extant bag collections, Vevers reworks and updates designs from the company's unique 160-year-old archive, thereby reinforcing signature Loewe styles. Working with the brand's Head of the Atelier, Vevers retains the company's traditional focus on craftsmanship without losing sight of what works in today's market. The energy of Madrid consistently informs Vevers' work for Loewe. He is also inspired by the strong, sophisticated and groomed look of Spanish women – polished but sexy – a look which he refers to as 'provocative classicism'.

Jewellery designer Paloma Picasso, daughter of iconic artist Pablo Picasso, is a favourite muse of Vevers – she even has a Loewe bag named in her honour.

Although the brand also includes apparel, Loewe are considered an authority on accessories, which is the definite focus of the label. Characteristics of the Loewe accessories range include a mix of exotic skins such as lizard, snake and ostrich, as well as the use of hardware as decoration. The Spring/Summer 09 bag collection boasts shapes with a distinctive, grown-up feel to them and features slouchy hobos, neat satchels and camera bags. Hardware is key, with decorative rope effects, padlocks and military buttons appearing throughout the collection.

The Calle bag (calle means street in Spanish) is inspired by supermarket carrier bags. This sack-shaped bag is made from beautiful soft leather and detailed with metallic trim and a metal hardware lock. An upgraded luxury version of the everyday shopper, the Calle bag takes the ordinary and makes it extraordinary.

A key archive piece that Vevers has revisited is the Amazona bag. Originally designed by Dario Rossi in 1975, the year Spanish dictator Franco died, this piece represented a new time and freedom when it was first released. With its rounded-off rectangular shape, structured handles and miniature padlock, the Amazona now comes in a selection of different colourways and skins.

The Amazona is an endlessly versatile bag – sumptuous leather versions with Loewe's logo depicting four interlinked 'L's are the height of classic chic, while blue paint-splattered ponyskin versions channel a casual, contemporary cool. At more than 30 years old, the Amazona has a longevity that makes it appeal to all generations, which in Vevers' eyes is the hallmark of a good bag. Vevers has said that he wants to bring back the soul of the Amazona bag, to make it famous. It could be said that this is what he has already achieved with the Loewe brand.

1 Detail from vintage Paloma bag, from Loewe archive.
2 Anagram embossed patent Fer bag, S/S 09. 3 Metallic Heritage satchels, S/S 09.
OVER THE PAGE (clockwise from left) Crocodile bag from Loewe archive, c.1960; Canvas Amazona weekender; Pink ostrich Calle, S/S 09; Storm Paint Splash haircalf Amazona bag; Truffle ostrich Calle Hobo 40 bag.

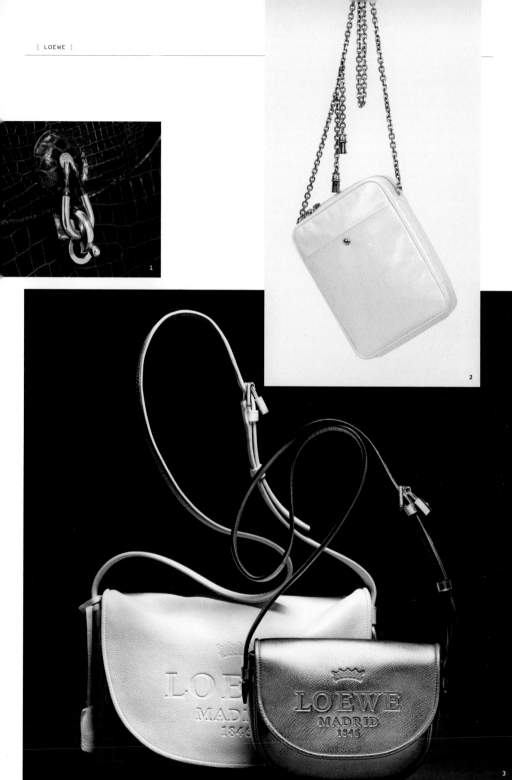

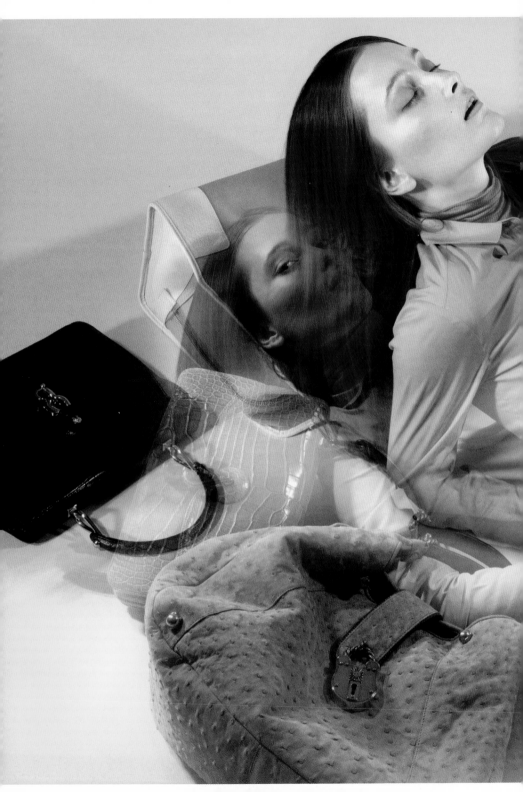

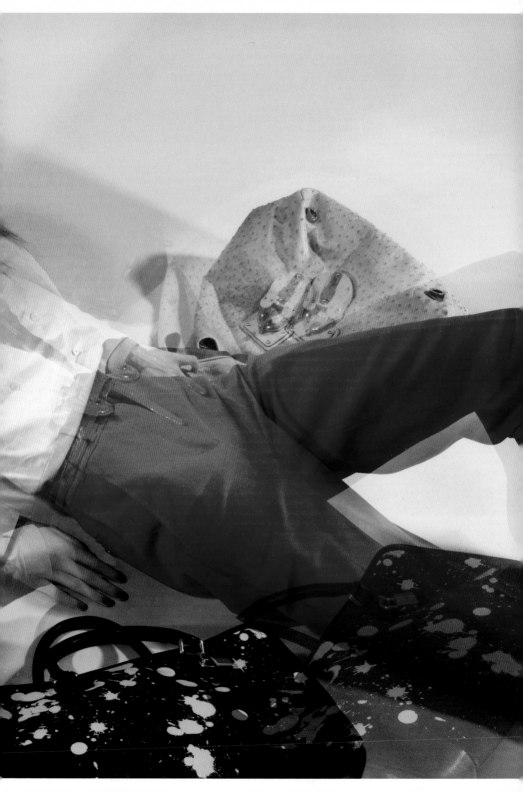

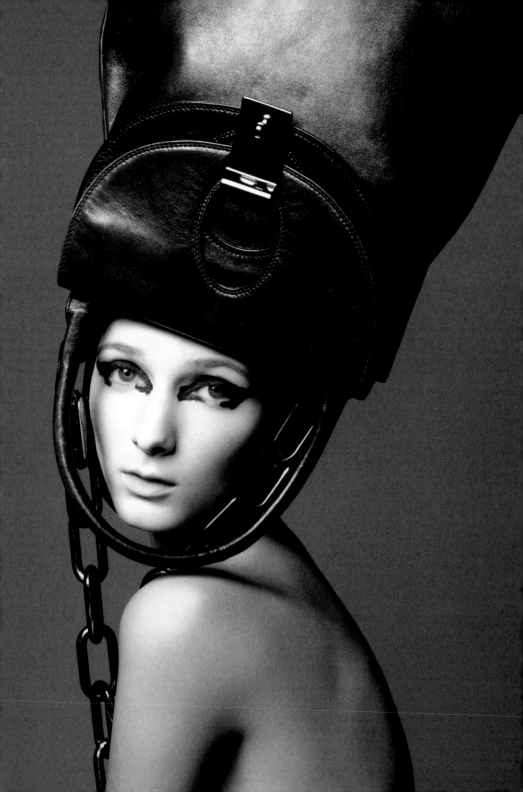

America's darling of fashion, Marc Jacobs
has an ability to design instinctively,
capturing the imagination of the fashion
world by delivering pieces that convey a
love of fashion and a commitment to quality.

MARC
JACOBS

OPPOSITE Blue Daydream tote, A/W 08/09.

Founded in 1986
www.marcjacobs.com

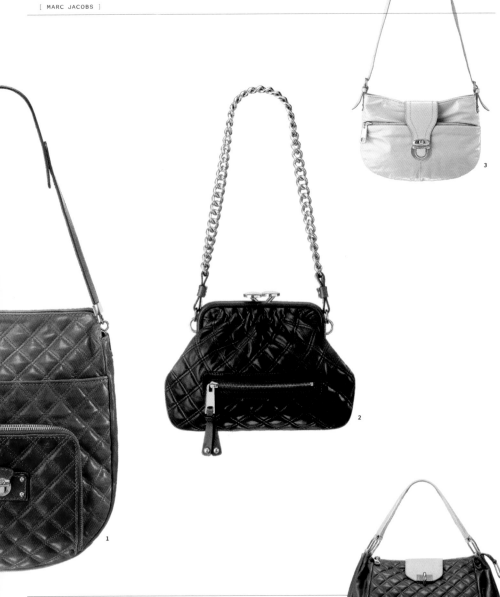

1 Brown Hobo, A/W 08/09. 2 Purple mini Stam, A/W 05/06.
3 Ivory small shoulder bag, S/S 04. 4 True Blue, A/W
08/09. 5 Metallic blue Stam, A/W 05/06. 6 Ivory East/
West tote, S/S 05. 7 Honeydew small Georgie, S/S 06.

MARC JACOBS IS UNQUESTIONABLY ONE OF THE MOST RENOWNED AND TALKED ABOUT DESIGNERS OF THE LAST TWO DECADES.

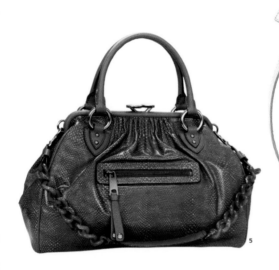

5

6

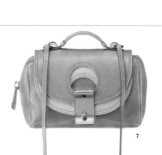

7

The youngest ever designer to be awarded the fashion industry's highest tribute, the Council of Fashion Designers of America's Perry Ellis Award for new fashion talent, Marc Jacobs has achieved more than most since graduating from the Parsons School of Design in 1984. Starting out designing hand-knit sweaters for the Weiser Family's chain of Charivari stores, Jacobs launched his own collection in 1986. Jacobs has since been recognized by the CFDA as 'Designer of the Year' on five occasions – womenswear in 1992 and 1997, menswear in 2002, and accessories in 1999 and 2003.

1995 saw the launch of Jacobs' first full collection of men's ready-to-wear. Based upon what he wanted to have in his own wardrobe, this collection propelled Jacobs into the spotlight, being both accessible and wearable – two important qualities that he continues to apply to all his collections and accessories lines.

In 1997 Jacobs, along with long-time collaborator Robert Duffy, was appointed by Louis Vuitton. As Artistic Director, Jacobs works on many of the house's collections, including men's and women's ready-to-wear lines, small leather goods and handbags. It is this experience that has laid the foundations for the Marc Jacobs brand we know today.

By working for a luxury house whose philosophy is also focused on quality, Jacobs was able to explore and merge quality with a love for fashion without compromising on either. The resulting experience resulted in the launch of his first handbag collection in 2000.

Inspired by 1950s' frame bags, vintage and elegance are the themes that run throughout each season's collections. It was the Stam bag that placed Marc Jacobs handbags firmly on the arm of the world's most fashionable women. Named after model Jessica Stam, who inspired Marc during his Autumn/Winter 05/06 collection, Jacobs played with amplified features such as the frame and kiss lock closure in the creation of this bag. Combined with quilted leather and a metal chain strap, Jacobs developed a must-have style in the Stam bag. The designer also created the exclusive Classic Stam bag, a reinterpreted version of the original that he offers in new materials, colours and hardware options each season.

Celebrity endorsements are a major component of the Marc Jabobs empire, and Jacobs himself has become a celebrity on the New York scene. His fashion shows have become as much about the front row celebrity audience as the collection itself.

Many compare the Stam bag to the Hermès Birkin and CHANEL 2.55 bags, and thus place the Stam bag central to the most recent rise of the IT bag. Not unlike Hermès, Jacobs affectionately names all of his bags after his friends, collaborators and those who have inspired him. While the handbag line has soared in popularity, the collections continue to maintain Jacobs' singular style and sophistication, without being distracted by changing trends.

Jacobs has an inherent ability to instinctively create what his adoring fans covet every season. The most talked about Jacobs bag for Spring/Summer 08 was the Bruna bag, while the Robert Jennifer bag (Autumn/Winter 08/09) is likely to become a bestseller.

Jacobs may have dropped the gloss and veneer of his earlier collections, but the same note of determination and drive for edginess continues to amaze. Nothing is too risky for Jacobs. Besides his main ready-to-wear lines for men and women, Jacobs has successfully launched diffusion line 'Marc by Marc Jacobs', children's line 'Little Marc' and more recently a homeware range in conjunction with Waterford. An unprecedented success story, Marc Jacobs is one of the most important designers of his generation.

OPPOSITE Purple quilted mini Stam, A/W 08/09.

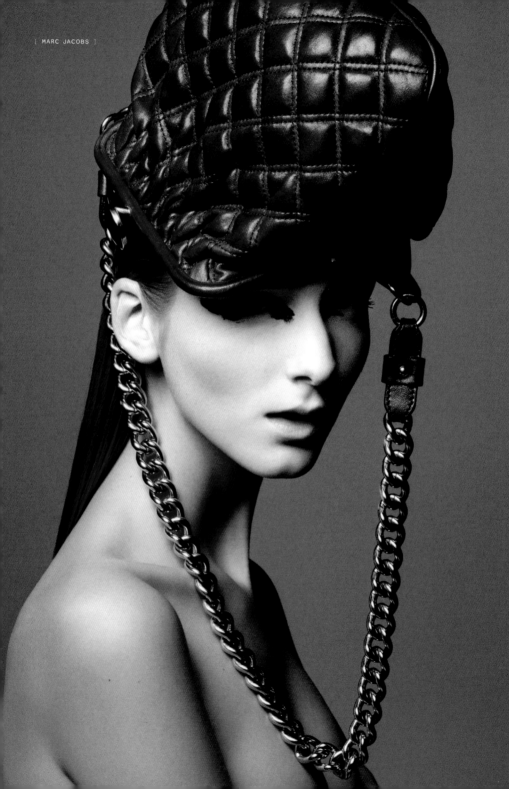

MOSCHINO

Established in 1983, Moschino continues
to employ fun and frivolity in the name
of fashion after more than a quarter of
a century in the business.

OPPOSITE Absolutely Lovely bag, S/S 08.

Founded in 1983
www.moschino.com

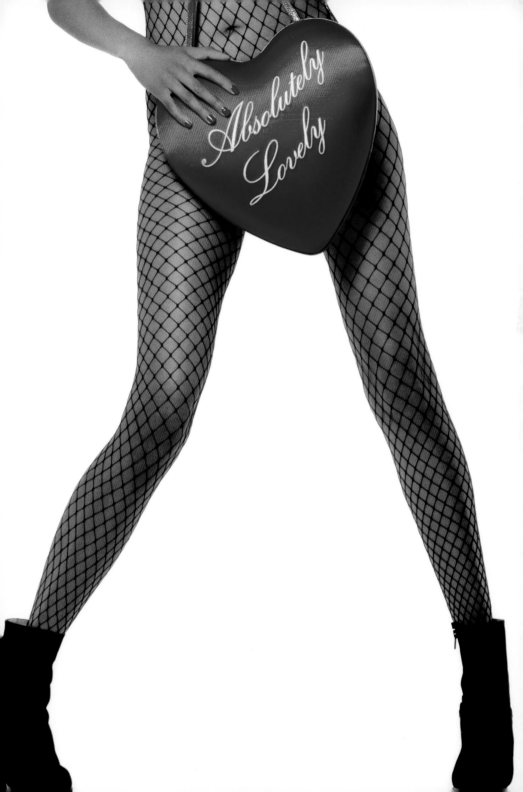

NOBODY DOES PLAYFUL, QUIRKY, HUMOROUS AND FEMININE BETTER THAN MOSCHINO

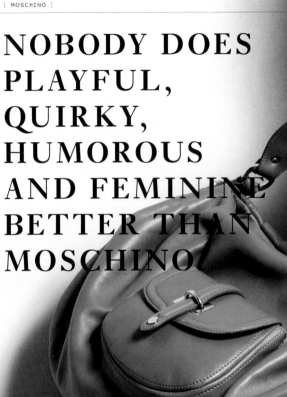

1,2&3 Moschino S/S 09 pre-collection. **4&5** Moschino collection, S/S 09.

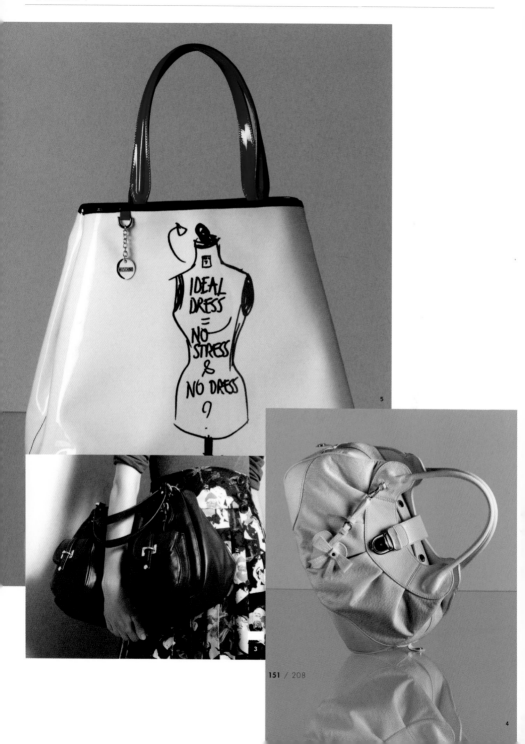

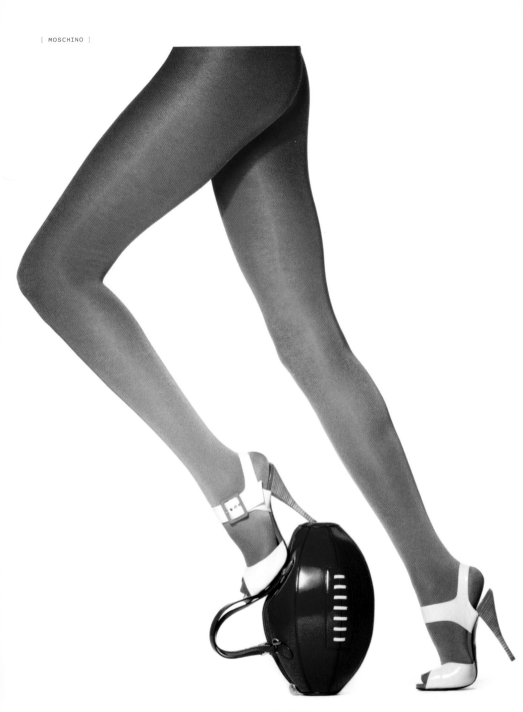

Credit for the continued playful ethos of the Moschino brand is due to Creative Director Rossella Jardini. Since taking over in 1994, Jardini has succeeded in retaining the founder's spirit and philosophical approach while introducing her own unique vision and expertise, having previously worked at some of Italy's most prestigious fashion houses including Bottega Veneta and Trussadi.

While Jardini has maintained the wit and charm of the brand, she has also moved away from the over-the-top gimmicks of the past and introduced a softer and more feminine aesthetic.

Moschino was created in 1983 by the late Franco Moschino, a designer famed for producing irreverent over-the-top designs that often challenged and provoked the fashion industry. A label known for its *classico con twist* (classic with a twist) style, Moschino bags are no exception.

'Moschino bags are recognizable for their quirky, ironic and playful styles as well as our more classic styles, all of which maintain the highest quality',

explains Rosella Jardini.

A mixture of extreme proportion and scale play a significant role in the design of the Moschino bag collections. Moschino also draws heavily on hardware, using it to personalize the bags:

'Metal hardware is always very important because it becomes the personalization of our bags, there are some seasons where the metal components are even more relevant as they become more decorative as well as functional.'

The heart, Moschino's longstanding signature symbol, has become the recurring motif that customers identify with the brand.

Jardini's approach to design always begins with colour, something she feels is particularly important in differentiating between each of the lines she works on.

'With all the collections I design, I always start from the colour palette, I use a general colour card, which I then divide between the various collections i.e., "Moschino", "Moschino Cheap and Chic", "Moschino Uomo" and ". ove Moschino". However, I never forget the value of classic tones when designing the bag collections.'

Jardini's approach to designing soft feminine bags is often determined by the leather she uses. Her preference is to work with soft-handled leathers such as nappa, patent and natural calfskin:

'I very rarely design rigid, stiff or structured bags. The inspiration for the bag's construction comes, first of all, from the materials that I decide to use and partly from the prêt-a-porter collection linked to the accessories.'

When she's researching a new collection, Jardini often delves into the Moschino archive, a wealthy source of design history spanning two decades. Now responsible for the image and style of all 20 clothing and accessories lines under the company's brands, as well as its advertising and store image, Jardini's achievements have much to contribute to the label's impressive history.

Over the past 25 years the brand has continually expanded and currently owns more than 20 different clothing and accessories lines including gloves, sunglasses, jewellery, ties, underwear, perfume and eyewear. In addition, Moschino boasts over 90 stores around the world in places as far reaching as St. Petersburg in Russia, Bangkok, Mumbai in India and Beijing as well as numerous dedicated spaces in some of the world's most prestigious department stores. Jardini's biggest project has been the design of Maison Moschino, a fairytale-themed boutique hotel expected to open in 2009 in Milan – yet another indication of the brand's impressive international positioning within the luxury market.

OPPOSITE Rugby Ball bag, Moschino A/W 98/99.

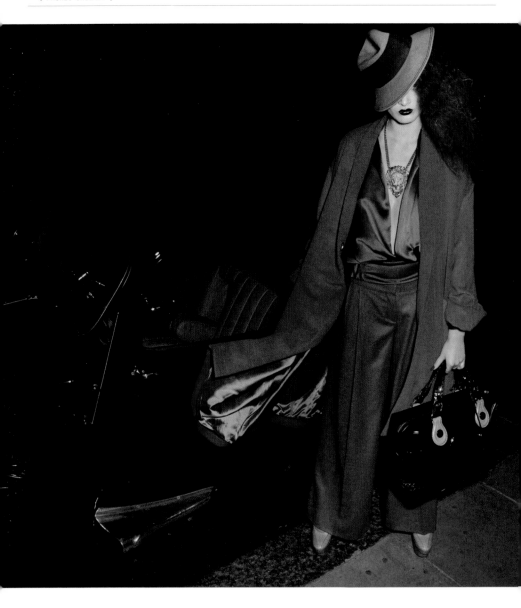

Pauric Sweeney's structural yet sleek designs combine unusual and daring materials to create luxury bags that are simply out of this world.

PAURIC SWEENEY

OPPOSITE Black patent Star bag.

Founded in 2005
www.pauricsweeneybags.com

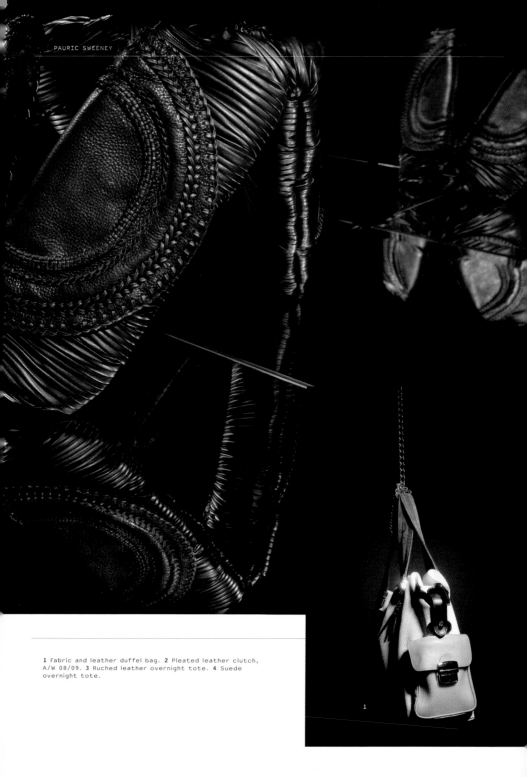

1 Fabric and leather duffel bag. 2 Pleated leather clutch,
A/W 08/09. 3 Ruched leather overnight tote. 4 Suede
overnight tote.

1

PAURIC SWEENEY DESIGNS BAGS FROM A DIFFERENT PERSPECTIVE THAN MOST.

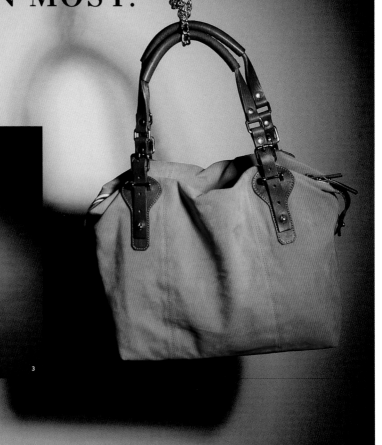

3

4

A former architecture student who designed furniture before moving on to fashion and accessories, Pauric Sweeney's inspirations range from music and literature to architecture and art theory.

When did you start designing bags?

'I began to design bags while I was presenting ready-to-wear collections and catwalks during London Fashion Week. I always showed accessories — whether they were intricately made head pieces, body accessories or jewellery. I moved into an accessories-only collection for Autumn/Winter 05 and it was embraced by press and buyers.'

Do you have a certain process when working on the collections?

'I work in a variety of ways, and am very process driven. From an initial aesthetic or theoretical viewpoint, I begin to assess and play with materials and hardware, and get to a sketch phase from which my sample makers and design team can work.'

Describe your techniques.

'I don't have a particular style — it really depends on the collection, materials I'm using and the sample makers I am working with. I tend to mix and combine materials that may not necessarily be used together normally.'

What is your signature design style?

'I am known for my classic 'Overnight' shape, which combines a very simple body shape with beautifully handcrafted woven leather handles made by an artisan in Umbria.'

What is it about your bags you are best known for?

'I think it's the daring and sometimes unexpected combinations of materials. In the Spring/Summer 2009 collection I combined perhaps 25 different materials in one particular bag.'

What inspires you and where do you find inspiration? Is there a theme that runs through each bag collection?

'I start with an idea and develop from there through sketches, mood boards, by listening to music and reading, looking at architecture... As this begins to take shape I add further ideas to find a harmony and balance in the collection.'

What materials and fabrications do you use?

'I use seemingly incompatible colours and textures such as iridescent python finishes and patent or matt leather contrasts ... new leather treatments which I develop with Tuscan tanneries, such as holographic leathers, lasered metallic finishes and quilted or embossed leathers and python. I always aim to create a distinctive and original feel for my materials palette. One season I used over 150 different materials in the collection. I enjoy seeing technical innovations combined with artisan techniques, a balance between tradition and modernity.'

Do you have a signature leather that you always use in your collection?

'My signature handle leather comes from an excellent tannery in Santa Croce sull'Arno (in Tuscany) that supplies soft shoulder leather. It is hand dyed using vegetable tanning processes, so is also kind to the environment. The material lasts a lifetime and beyond, it gets better the more you use it.'

How do you feel about the bag industry at the moment and how do you think it is going to develop in the future? Will customers be looking for a quick fix or something with longevity?

'I think customers are becoming increasingly discerning and sophisticated. Having said that, I don't think the answer lies in an either/or approach. Customers vary, and different attributes appeal to different needs.'

Do you have any thoughts on the IT bag? How would you define an IT bag?

'A bag that catches the zeitgeist and popular imagination. It is also a question of media focus and a certain buzz.'

Has the IT bag run its course?

'Bags can be a mirror to popular culture, there are great records that emerge and everyone catches the fever. In a similar sense some iconic bags catch the mood of the moment and become popular... I don't think this will change.

OPPOSITE (left) Ryder Hobo bag in platinum python and leather; (right) Stingray clutch in graphite silver with chain.

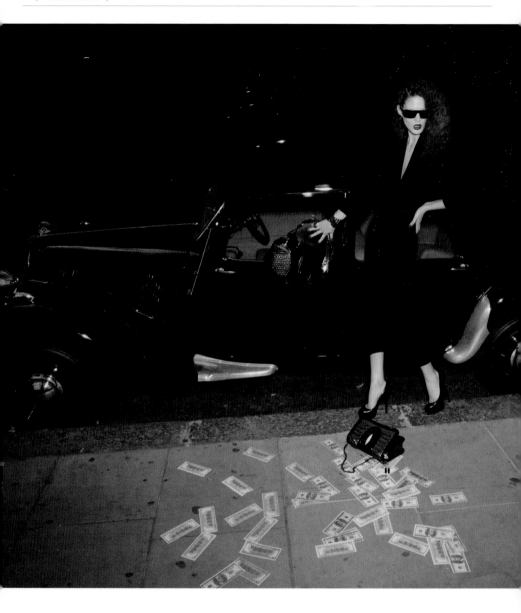

3.1 PHILLIP LIM

Phillip Lim's accessories, like his apparel lines, are classic yet at the same time individual. His design ethos is to create beautiful bags with a touch of madness.

OPPOSITE (from top to bottom) Selection from A/W 08/09; spotted bag, S/S 09; blue tote, Resort 2007.

Founded in 2005
www.31philliplim.com

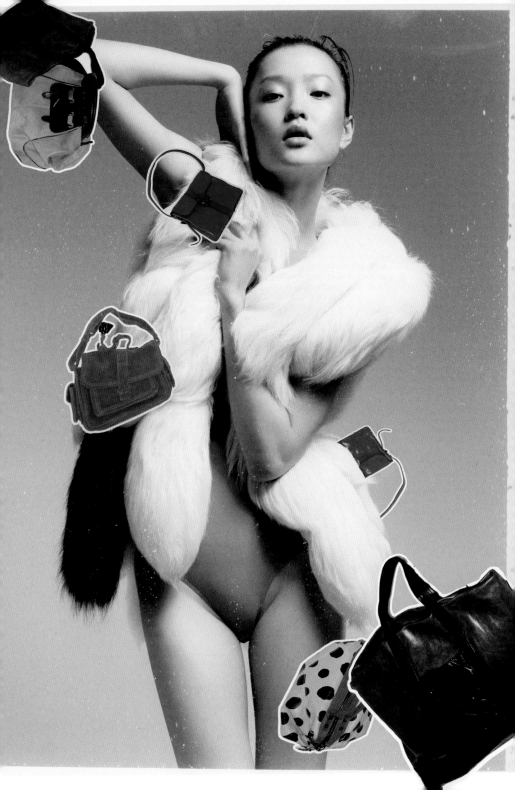

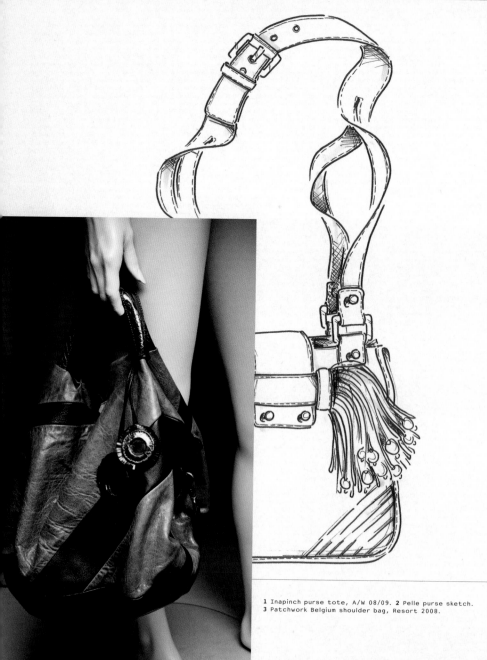

1 Inapinch purse tote, A/W 08/09. 2 Pelle purse sketch.
3 Patchwork Belgium shoulder bag, Resort 2008.

1

'OUR SIGNATURE
DESIGN STYLE IS
UNDERSTATED,
COOL AND
MULTI-FUNCTIONAL'

Having only launched his eponymous 3.1 Phillip Lim collection with partner Wen Zhou in 2005, Phillip Lim's achievements have been nothing short of impressive. The brand is already represented in 45 countries and available at nearly 400 stores, boutiques and department stores worldwide. Stylish, elegant and effortlessly cool, Phillip Lim is enjoying international success at the highest level.

How did you initially get into bag design?

'It was an organic and obvious choice to have bags to accompany the collection, a further extension of the 3.1 aesthetic. My background is in garments, so accessories have been a fun and exciting new learning process.'

Do you have a certain working process? If so, which part do you enjoy the most?

'Designing accessories is a process that I refer to as micro designing; it's similar to designing a car, there is a lot of time spent on small details within the framework of the bigger picture. Bags have to be great functionally as well as aesthetically. My favourite part of designing bags is attempting to marry all of these elements and have them work well together.'

Describe the type of constructions you use for your bags.

'3.1 bags are based on the idea of soft structure and classic shapes. There is always a "slouch" aesthetic to our bags. I like the idea that no two bags look the same. We also like to experiment with different treatments, leathers and construction techniques. We revolve our bag collections around the kinds of bags that we like to carry ourselves and there is always a 3.1 twist; classic with a sense of madness.'

What is your signature design style?

'It is understated, cool and multi-functional. The Tally bag has been a favourite among the 3.1 girls. I love this bag because of the drape of the lamb leather and the subtle detailing. This bag was based on a combination of the hobo and classic carpetbag. I love big bags — they're such a statement without being obnoxious. I like how confident girls are that carry big bags.'

Where do you find you inspiration?

'I like looking at vintage garments and jewellery, I am a huge fan of Native American pieces and their intricate designs and handiwork and I could also never tire of jewellery from the Art Deco period.'

Do you have any designer favourites or heroes that you like and admire?

'I have a lot of respect for Stella McCartney and her ability to create really great looking accessories using alternative materials.'

What materials and fabrics do you use, and is hardware important?

'I use all kinds of materials for the collection. It just has to be the right look and the right feel. We have used everything from washed lamb-, goat-, pony- and calfskin to Teflon-coated canvases. We usually mix up the materials on the bags to create a graphic look. I like to work with leathers that have a nice weight and drape to them, to create the slouchy look. Hardware can improve the look of a bag tremendously, however I don't think all bags require it.'

How do you feel about the bag industry?

'I think it's a very exciting time for bag designers, there is a demand for bags and the consumers are much more sophisticated in what they want their bags to do and what they look like.'

Do you have any thoughts on the so-called IT bag?

'I think good press has a huge hand in an IT bag. I don't think it has run its course, however I don't think there is the same kind of frenzy as there was, when the term "IT bag" was first coined. There are so many good designers out there making great bags, how can we possibly give all our attention to one bag?'

OPPOSITE 1 Tally bag, S/S 09. 2 Domino handbag, S/S 09. 3 Kanvas tote, S/S 09. 4 Heloise pouch, S/S 09. OVER THE PAGE (top left) striped bag S/S 09; (top right) camera bag, Resort 2007; selected other bags from A/W 08/09 collection.

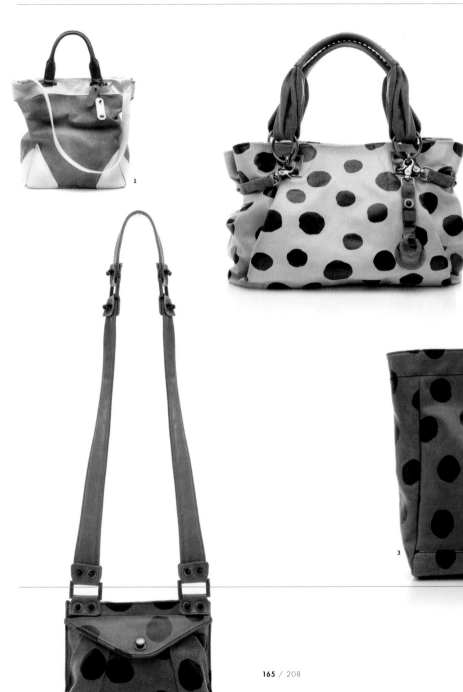

1

2

3

4

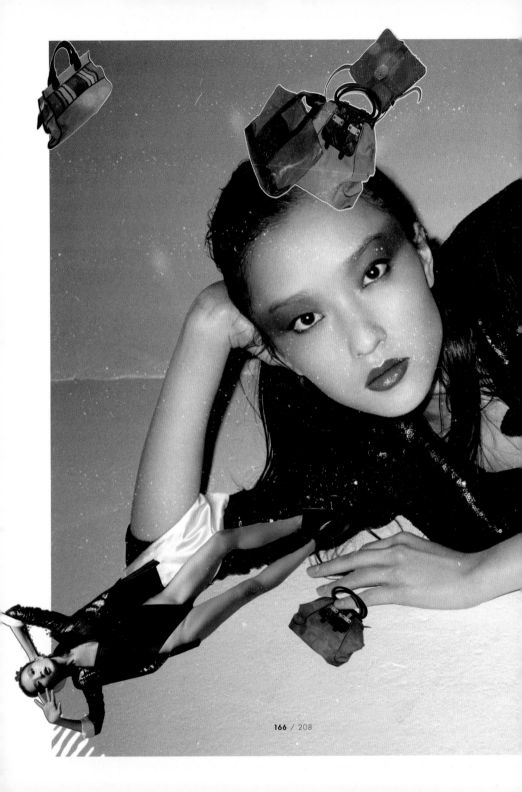

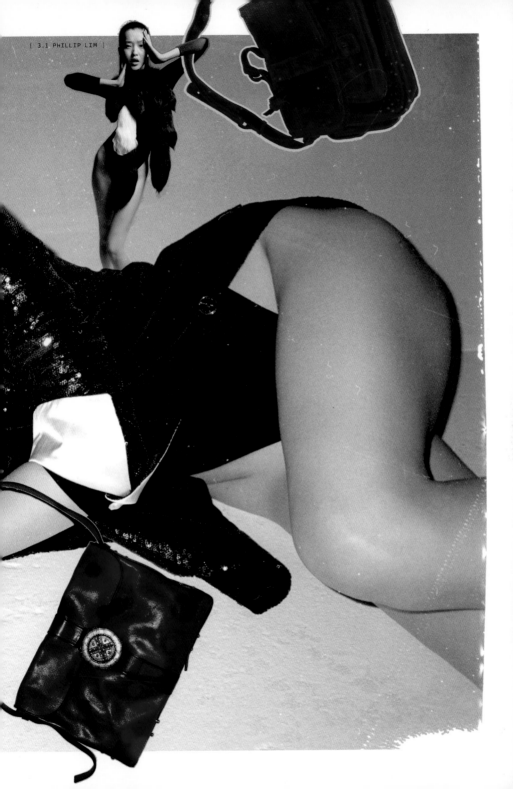

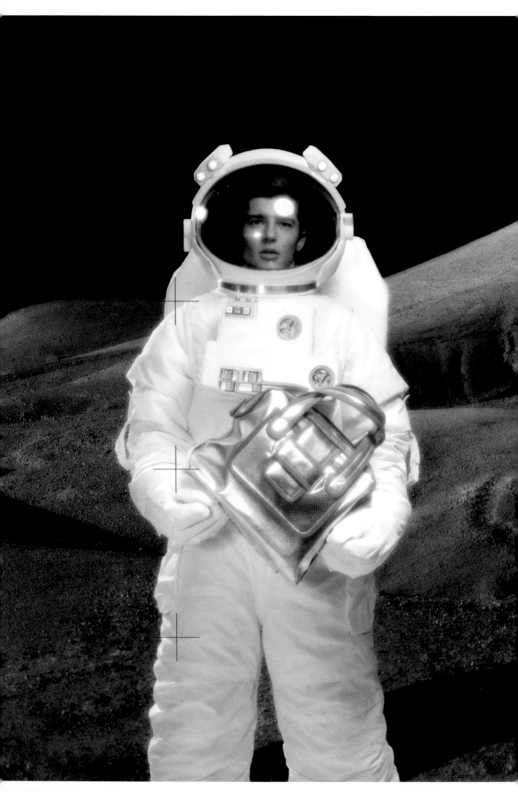

Unquestionably one of fashion's leading luminaries, Pierre Hardy is also one of the most accomplished luxury accessories designers in the world.

PIERRE HARDY

OPPOSITE Handbag in perforated nappa and suede leather, S/S 09.

Founded in 1999
www.pierrehardy.com

BOLD AND BEAUTIFUL, THE PIERRE HARDY BAG IS INSTANTLY RECOGNIZABLE BY ITS STATEMENT USE OF GRAPHICS AND DARING COLOUR SCHEMES.

1

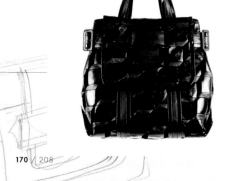

2

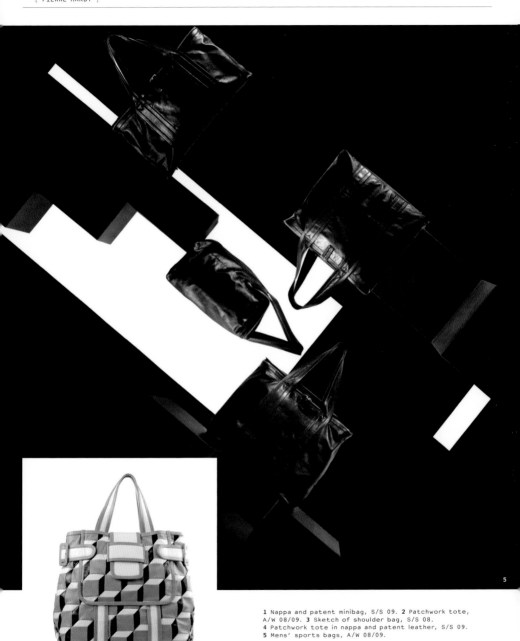

1 Nappa and patent minibag, S/S 09. 2 Patchwork tote,
A/W 08/09. 3 Sketch of shoulder bag, S/S 08.
4 Patchwork tote in nappa and patent leather, S/S 09.
5 Mens' sports bags, A/W 08/09.

After studying fine art and painting, Pierre Hardy went on to design footwear at the prestigious French haute couture house of Christian Dior in 1988 before becoming Head of Design at the quintessentially French luxury brand Hermès. In 2002, he joined Balenciaga as Head Designer for the footwear line.

Pierre Hardy launched his critically acclaimed footwear collection in 1999 and continued his success with the launch of his bag collection in 2007.

While Hardy may be primarily associated with footwear, he has wasted little time in establishing his bags as the designer must-have in a hugely competitive market. All of this in less than three years, and not a logo or sign of aggressive branding in sight.

Pierre Hardy's design process always begins with a sketch – the part of the process he enjoys the most. Avoiding references to fashion history and trends in his collections, Hardy instead prefers to draw inspiration from the things he finds beautiful. Objects, the arts, architecture such as the Memphis Design Group and conceptual artists such as Daniel Buren and Pol Bury have inspired Hardy's various collections.

Femininity is something Hardy strives to express in his work. However, the designer takes an ambiguous approach, mixing traditional feminine values with strength and masculinity to create a modern twist. While Hardy's designs are undoubtedly modern they are also great examples of simplicity, and his strengths lie not only in his great ideas but also in his ability to employ those without exaggerating them:

'I love clean lines and sculptural shapes and try to simplify the design to an essence.'

The initial idea for the Pierre Hardy bag collection was to create something very different to anything else that was on the market (in contrast to his approach to the Hardy footwear collection). He believes that

'The Pierre Hardy bag collection is a game of contrasts, the contrast between strong design and the suppleness of the materials and imposing volumes and the lightness of the bags.'

Hardy's bag designs playfully juxtapose soft sensual shapes and constructions with bold linear appliqué:

'The contrast trim traces the contours and the details of the bags, just like a sketch on paper'.

Hardy's purist approach to design comes as a breath of fresh air. Bold and beautiful, the Pierre Hardy bag is instantly recognizable by its statement use of graphics and daring colour schemes. Avoiding the use of distracting logos and unnecessary hardware, Hardy prefers to let the design speak for itself:

'I didn't want any useless, overweight hardware but instead wanted the focus to be on the leather trim that structures the bag.'

The Hardy mens' bag line is also based on the idea of design contrasts. Hardy brings a more subtle approach to this particular line, saying

'I wanted the bags to be soft but graphic, essential but with identity'.

Conceived as the accompaniment to his existing women's range, Hardy has yet again succeeded in creating a winning style that appeals to the modern consumer.

With no limit to his successes, Pierre Hardy's achievements have confirmed the designer's reputation as both a skilled craftsman of leather goods and an innovative visionary talent within the fashion industry.

Maintaining his position at the pinnacle of modernity is something Hardy is extremely passionate about.

'I always try to bring something new to my designs but in the most radical way I can',

he explains. Created without bending to seasonal trends or historical fashion reference points, Hardy's unique vision is without doubt the secret to his success. Transcending time and place, his pieces are the epitome of great modern design.

OPPOSITE Clutch in 'perspective cubes' print leather, A/W 08/09.

172 / 208

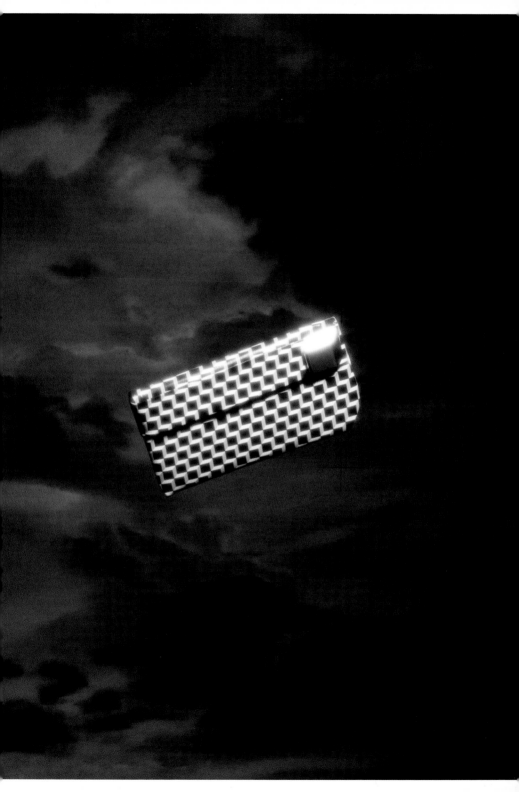

PORTS 1961

Sculpted works of art, Ports 1961 bags
transcend fashion fads with a unique and
inimitable style of their own, and are
perhaps most notable for their unexpected
use of materials.

OPPOSITE Hogni Clutch, N/63 collection, A/W 07/08.

Founded in 1961
www.ports1961.com

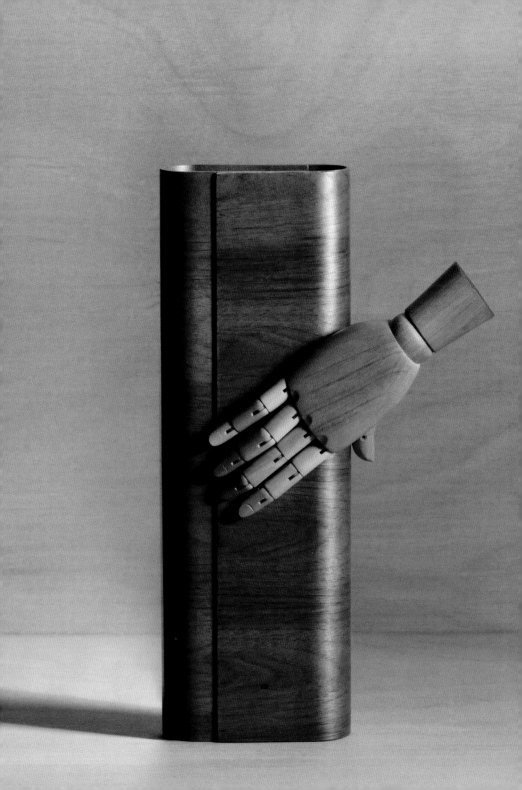

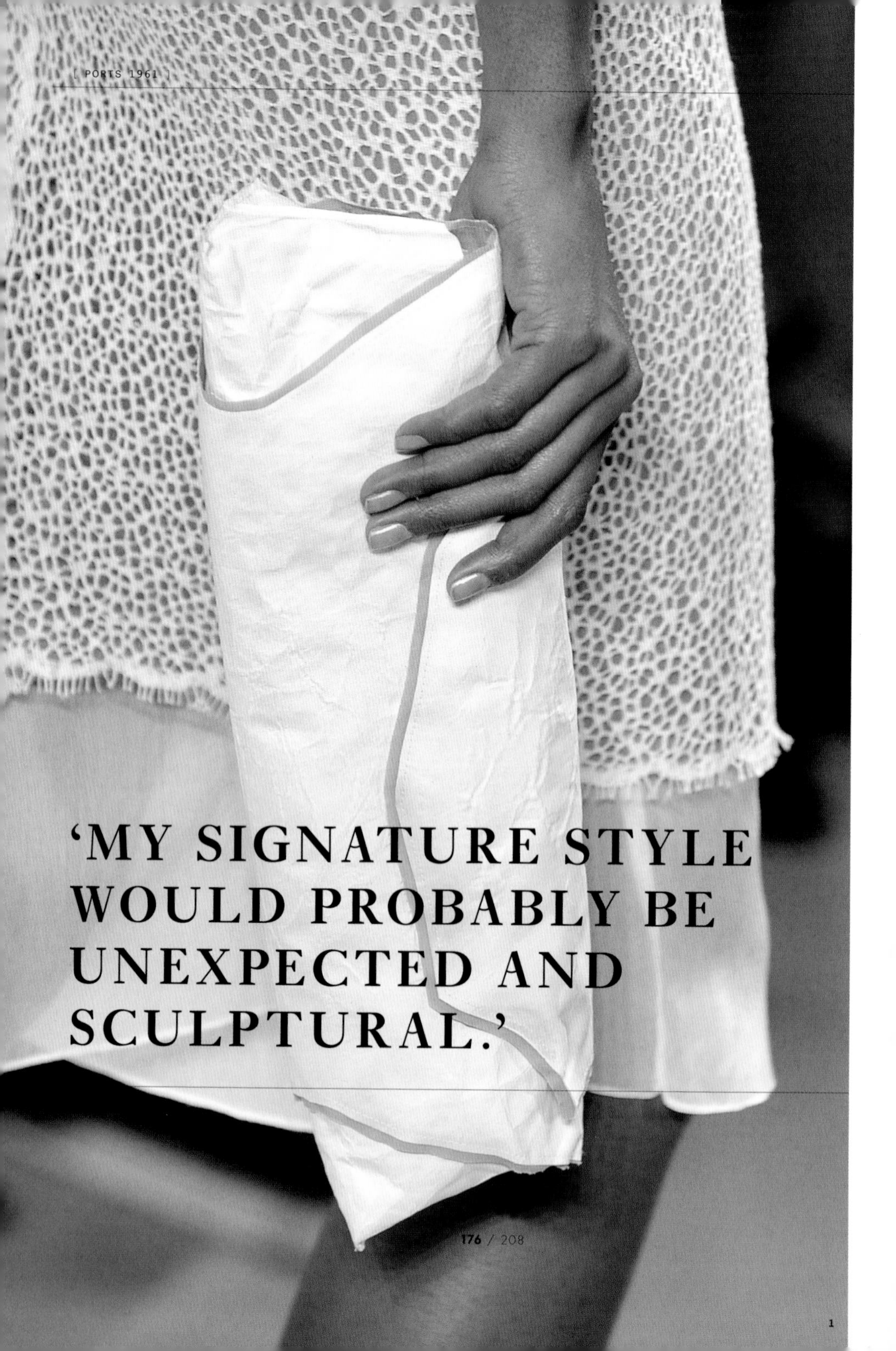

'MY SIGNATURE STYLE
WOULD PROBABLY BE
UNEXPECTED AND
SCULPTURAL.'

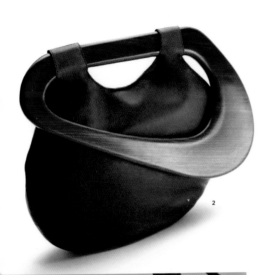

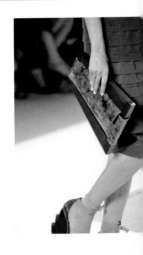

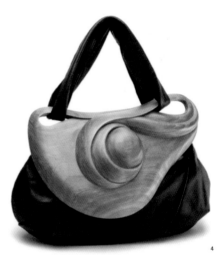

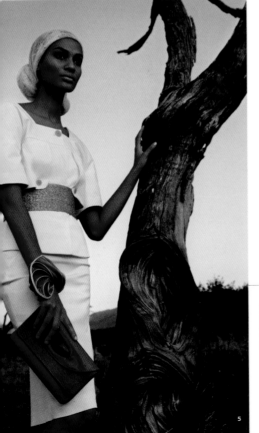

1 Osprey Roll Clutch, Beloved of the Sky collection, S/S
09. 2 Dair Wood Satchel, Lassair collection, A/W 08/09.
3 Major Yaku Clutch, Beloved of the Sky collection, S/S
09. 4 Edad Wood Messenger, Lassair collection, A/W
08/09. 5 Advertising campaign for Safari collection,
S/S 08.

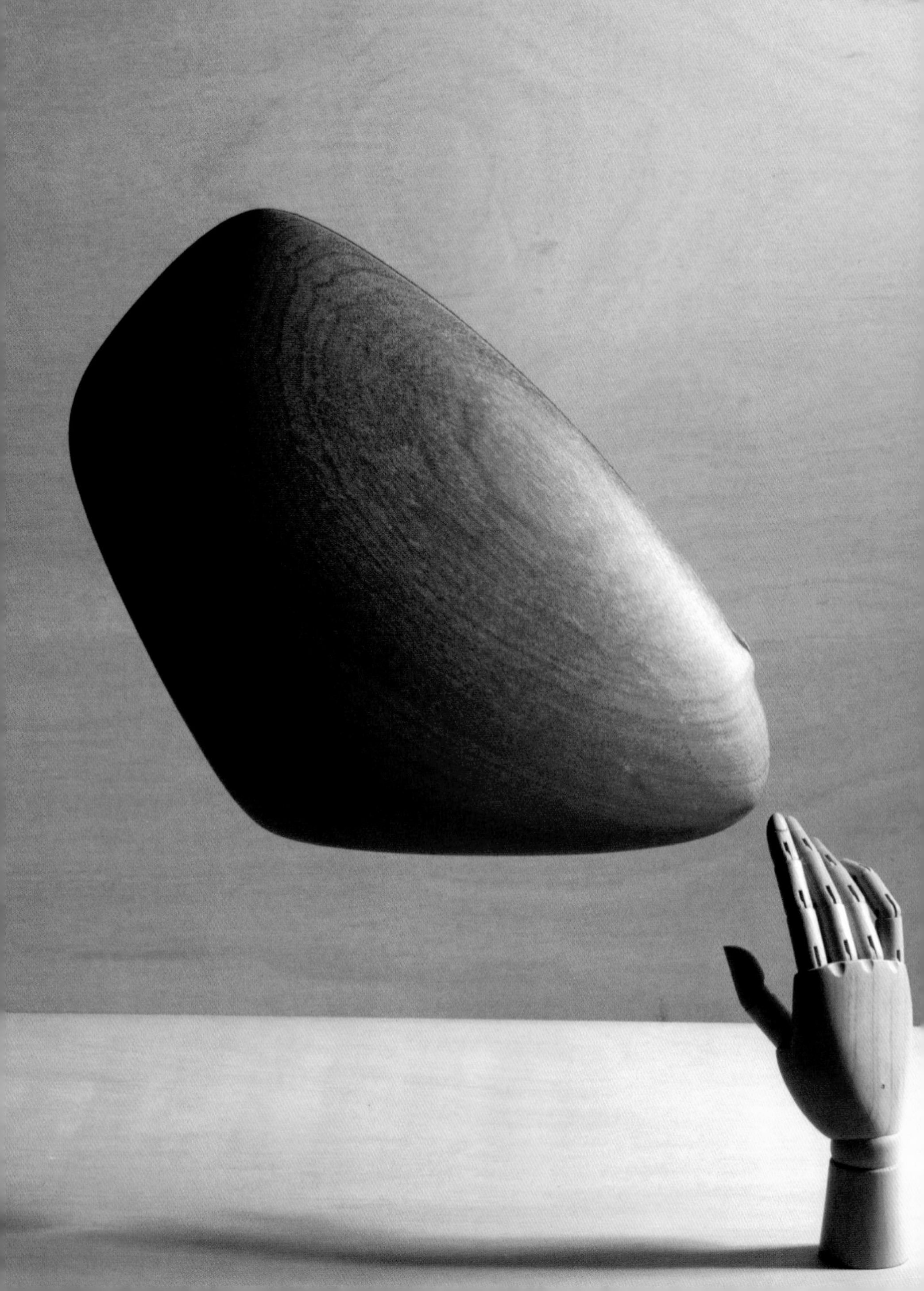

Launched in New York under the dynamic vision of Creative Director Tia Cibani, Ports 1961 combines high performance with a modern luxury aesthetic. Formerly known as Ports International, the brand was founded in 1961 and launched as a luxury sportswear line before changing hands in the early 1990s and re-launching in 2004.

When did you start designing bags?

'I have always been interested in accessories, and focused much more on them when I started presenting my ready-to-wear collection in New York. I just felt it was important to convey the whole message, to design the complete look with accessories, which would exist on a "real" day in a "real" woman's life.'

How did you initially get into bag design?

'I studied fashion design at Parsons in New York before joining the company. I never studied handbag construction or design, instead it found me in a very organic way when I had the idea to present a total look.'

Do you have a certain process when working on the collections, for example do you sketch first or make models of the bags?

'I usually begin with material and colour, I have a theme in mind and research it quite extensively. I think of key details I may like to incorporate into the bag, keeping in mind my inspiration as well as practicality. I then sketch shapes and consider the size and dimensions, as this will often have an affect on the details.'

How is your time divided on each part of the process?

'It is hard for me to say exactly, but I probably spend most of the time developing the bag technically. I work closely with the technician, keeping in mind the materials we have chosen and bringing it all together in a harmonious way. My favourite part of the process is working on the interior of the bag; I love designing the special details that feature on the inside.'

What type of bag constructions do you use and what are they inspired by?

'I guess that my signature construction would be my unexpected use of materials. I love to experiment and am not shy to try totally crazy detailing which often results in making the bag look like a piece of art. I have sculpted a solid piece of wood into a clutch bag before — that was fun!'

Describe your signature design style.

'I wouldn't call it sexy but certainly feminine and full of impact. I love oversized bags, exaggerated shapes and details, which make the bag more than just an essential item.'

What inspires you and where do you find your inspiration?

'Travel, and the people and cultures of all the places I encounter.'

Do you have any designer favourites or heroes, and what is it about them that you like and admire?

'My all-time favourite is Yves Saint Laurent, the original, he's legendary, an icon. I totally admire him for shaping modern fashion as we know it today.'

Are you planning to expand your business by introducing new lines and collections?

'My future plans include expanding my bag collection into travel gear.'

How do you think the industry is going to develop in the future? Will customers be looking for a quick fix, or something with longevity?

'I think that longevity is always key. I love all of my bags and that's because I purchased them with emotion. I feel that, essentially, that is what a woman wants to feel — a special emotion for the investment she makes. This way she will treasure her bags forever.'

How would you define an IT bag? Is there still room for it or has it run its course?

'An IT bag is the right bag at the right time worn in the right place by the right girl. I think that so many factors play a role in creating an IT bag. It's no longer just about the bag itself, there is always room for it and I definitely don't think it has run its course.'

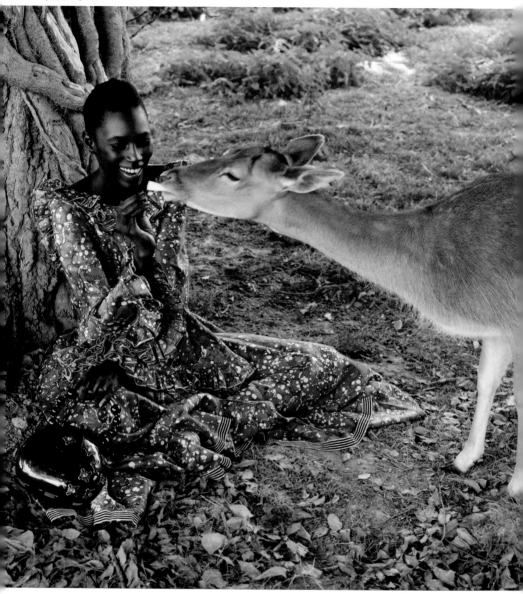

ROCIO

A world away from artificial and mundane materials, UK label Rocio prides itself on creating exquisite, handcrafted collector's pieces out of sustainable acacia wood.

OPPOSITE A classic shaped Rocio handbag in a lacquered dark green finish embossed with flowers.

Founded in 2006
www.rociobags.com

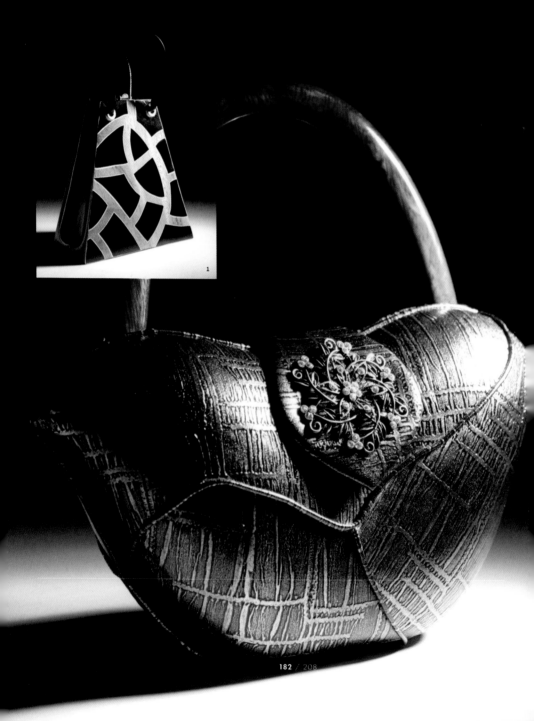

'OUR BAGS ARE UNIQUE, NOT ONLY IN THE MATERIAL FROM WHICH THEY ARE MADE, BUT IN THE DESIGN STYLE THEY POSSESS. VINTAGE SHAPES INFUSED WITH CHIC MODERN ELEMENTS, THE BAGS TAKE A CLASSIC AESTHETIC AND GIVE IT A MODERN TWIST'

1 The Ramesses, 2007. 2 The Rainier, 2007, enveloped in satin with Swarovski crystal feature. 3 The Honey, 2006.

3

Rocio is a luxury brand with a difference. It may specialize in handmade designs, but these are no ordinary designer handbags. Made from sustainably sourced acacia wood, Rocio bags are beautifully crafted works of art that prove that being environmentally aware doesn't have to come at the cost of being stylish.

Rocio was established in Scotland in 2006 by Rocio Olbes and Hamish Menzies, with the objective of returning fashion to the sphere of the arts. Entirely handmade and embellished or inlaid with gemstones, exotic skins and fine leathers, each Rocio bag can take from six to eight weeks to complete. Here, Rocio Olbes explains the ethos behind the brand.

How did you initially begin designing bags?

'I have always been artistic, so designing accessories seemed like a natural progression. It was finding a material as unique as sustainable acacia wood that was the difficult part. In order for our label to be recognized in an industry as fast-paced and quickly changing as the fashion world, we needed to launch something that was totally and utterly unique, something that would gain us notoriety without sacrificing fierce fashion style and practical qualities.'

Describe your techniques.

'I always begin with a simple pencil sketch, trying to capture the image or design in my head before developing it further. I also believe that as you grow so do your techniques, and you also develop new ones along the way. I am constantly changing and exploring, but have not yet developed any particular method or technique that I am set on.'

What inspires you?

'I find inspiration in so much: when I travel, to be engrossed in different cultures and see how the colour hues of every country are so unique; I find inspiration in the people around me and their natural style; in the style icons from the past, such as Audrey Hepburn, Grace Kelly, Twiggy and Bridget Bardot — all immortal in their own way, each one changing the course of the fashion world and redefining what it is to be an icon; I find inspiration in the designs of the maestros of our industry, such as Karl Lagerfeld, Valentino, Yves Saint Laurent, each reinterpreting fashion, and in how they have continually created the most beautiful designs the world has ever seen. All of these inspire me not only as a designer, but also as a fashion lover.'

What materials and fabrications do you use?

'Rocio designer bags are strictly handmade from the finest selection of sustainable acacia wood. These works of art are cut and finished to perfection. They vary from bags with an elegant natural finish to those incorporating lavish materials such as snakeskin, leathers, gems, crystals, paints and carvings.'

What are your plans and ambitions for the future?

'I believe you never cross the finish line. There is always something new, or something new to create. My visions for the brand are set — expanding our label as a global luxury brand.'

How do you feel about the accessories industry, and how do you think it's going to develop in the future?

'I feel the accessories industry, like the rest of the fashion world, is changing. Not only in style, but in what the customer desires. The world is going "green", and everyone has become extremely environmentally aware. I think it is a challenge for luxury labels such as us to come up with products and designs that do not sacrifice one inch of style but are environmentally aware. We have created a line that is environmentally safe, but that is extremely fashionable. I believe that it is such an important issue, and the fashion world is changing because of it. Before anything else we must take care of our planet, because without our planet there is no future.'

MAIN PICTURE The Audrey, 2007. **INSET** The Chequer, 2007.
OVER THE PAGE Collette bag.

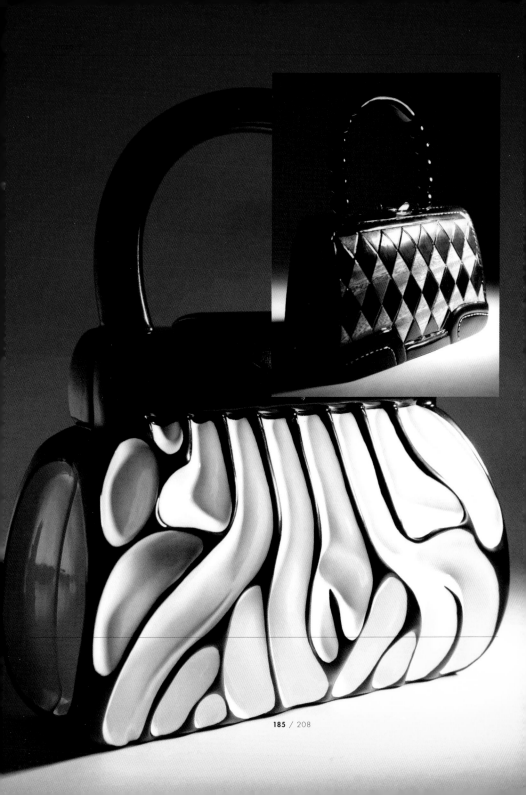

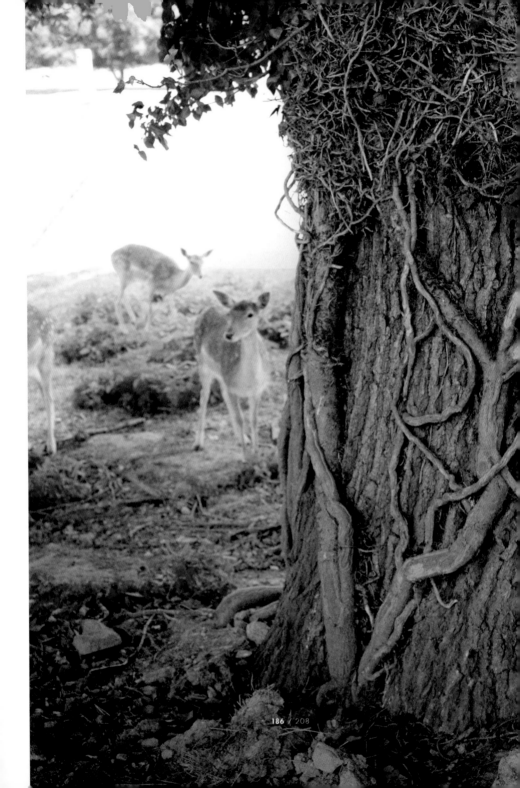

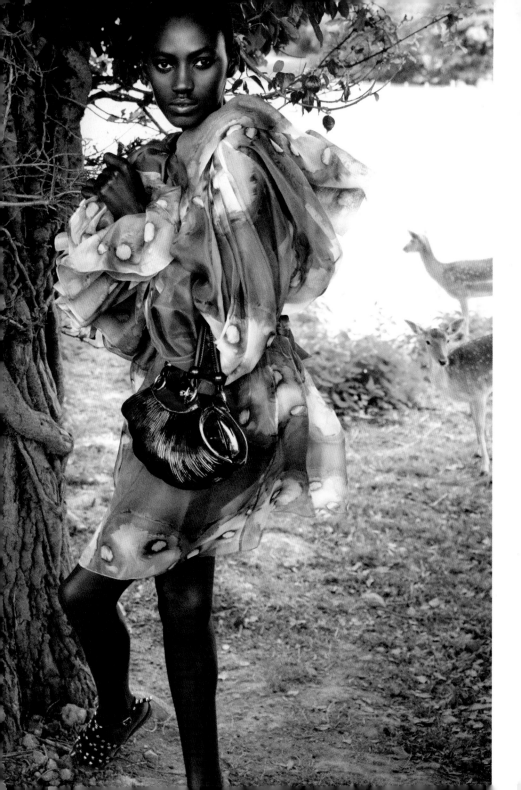

VERSACE

Versace handbags, along with the rest of
the accessories range, are coveted for
their ability to transform an outfit into
a grand fashion statement.

OPPOSITE Patent leather bag, A/W 08/09.

Founded in 1978
www.versace.com

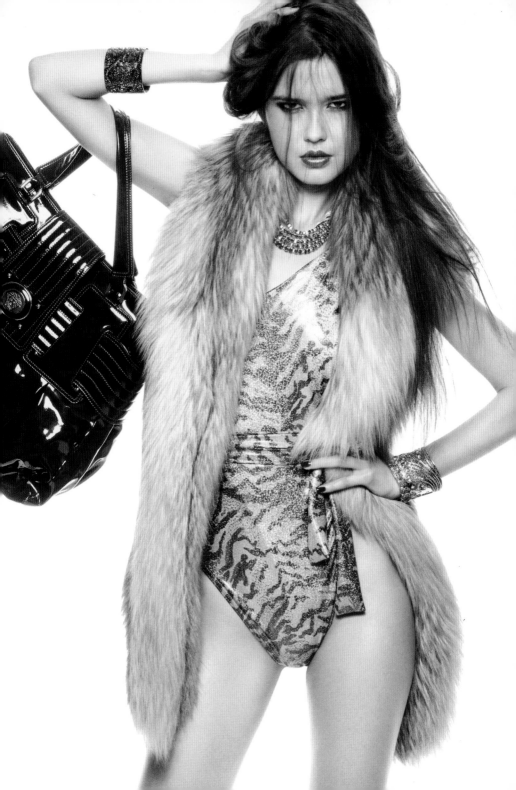

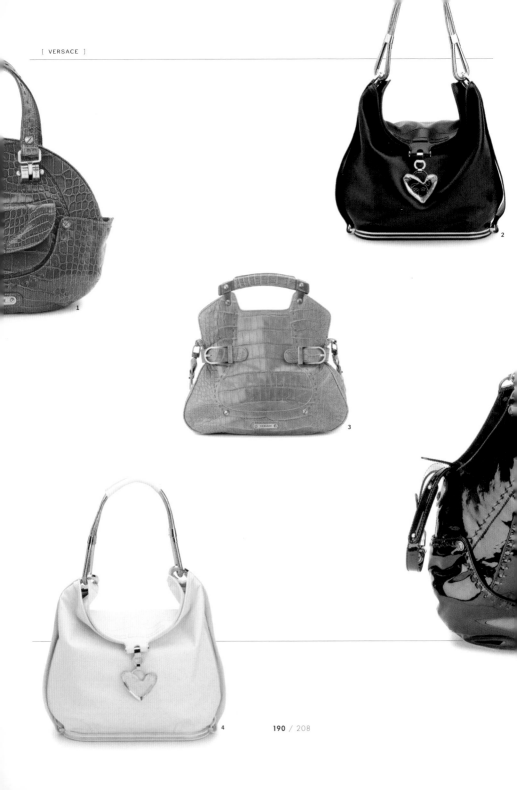

THE DISTINCT VERSACE STYLE IS SYNONYMOUS WITH STATEMENT DRESSING AND SUMPTUOUS DESIGNS OF BOLD COLOURS AND MATERIALS.

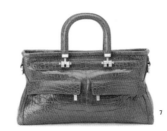

1 Soul Bag, A/W 08/09. 2 Heart-detail Bag, S/S 09.
3 Jewel Bag, A/W 08. 4 Heart-detail Bag, S/S 09. 5 Kiss
Bag A/W 08/09. 6 Studded tassel-detail Bag, S/S 09.
7 Luxe Bag, A/W 08/09. 8 S/S 09.

In addition to being one of the world's most recognized fashion houses, the Versace brand has become a global symbol for Italian luxury. The distinctive Versace style is synonymous with dressing for drama in sumptuous designs of bold colours and precious materials. But the Versace label may be most well-known for its sheer ability to defy scale and court celebrity.

Gianni Versace started his career as a costume designer at the Teatro della Scala before founding his first boutique in Milan in 1978. The decadent style and irreverent rock-star attitude of the Versace brand had an immediate impact on the fashion world. The brand's insignia, which features a Medusa head and Greek key, was selected because of Gianni's fascination with Greek mythology and architecture. Gianni also felt that the mythical figure of Medusa was appropriate for the Versace brand because he wanted his designs to evoke the same goddess-like qualities and provocative responses that Medusa did.

Given the philosophy behind its insignia, it is no surprise that the Versace brand is unequivocally linked to the world of celebrity. These celebrities act both as clients and as 'faces' – or models – for the house. Indeed, the rise of the supermodel is in part a result of Gianni's vision for his brand in that everything had to be larger than life. In the summer of 1991, Gianni showed his Spring/Summer 92 collection using the four most famous models of that time: Cindy Crawford, Linda Evangelista, Naomi Campbell and Tatjana Patitz. This ongoing relationship with celebrity culture has ensured that Versace has a longstanding audience with celebrities such as Elton John, Beyoncé, Madonna, Jennifer Lopez and Liz Hurley – and all of their fans.

Following its founders death, the brand has recently repositioned itself under the guidance of Creative Director Donatella Versace, who is also the company's Vice President.

Recognizing the changing attitudes of its clients, Versace has toned-down its high gloss aesthetic and replaced it with a more simplistic chic style. The handbag line maintains the glamour of the Versace name, but there is also more emphasis on understated luxury: logos are subtly embossed rather than heavily emblazoned, and bags that once screamed opulence have given way to classic, elegant styles such as the Kayla Hobo. Versace continues to create desirable pieces that reflect the lifestyles of modern women, which has helped build its reputation as a leading accessories brand.

Several Versace bags have become IT bags, which in turn have become overnight classics. The resurgent success of the Versace bag is a result of its ability to deliver both understated and exaggerated style. The Versace bag collection juxtaposes simple black leather clutches with metallic silver leather totes adorned with rhinestones, oversized 'V' logos and lavish brocade. While the variety in the collection attracts a continuous flow of new customers, maintaining the historical Versace aesthetic retains longstanding fans.

In a move that confirms Versace's ability to reinvent itself to appeal to new audiences, fashion designer Julie Verhoeven was commissioned to re-imagine the Versace iconography for its Spring/Summer 09 collection. The resulting glitz signals that the Versace glamour aesthetic has been retained in the accessories line, but there is also a sense of more fun now being had at Versace.

With over 80 boutiques across the globe, the Versace brand now includes everything from clothing, fragrances, cosmetics, accessories, home furnishings and, most recently, the fitting addition of the Versace Hotel and Spa – suitably named Palazzo Versace – on Australia's Gold Coast. Versace may have many imitators, but it's apparent that in both style and scale nothing can beat the real thing.

OPPOSITE Luxe Bag, A/W 08/09.

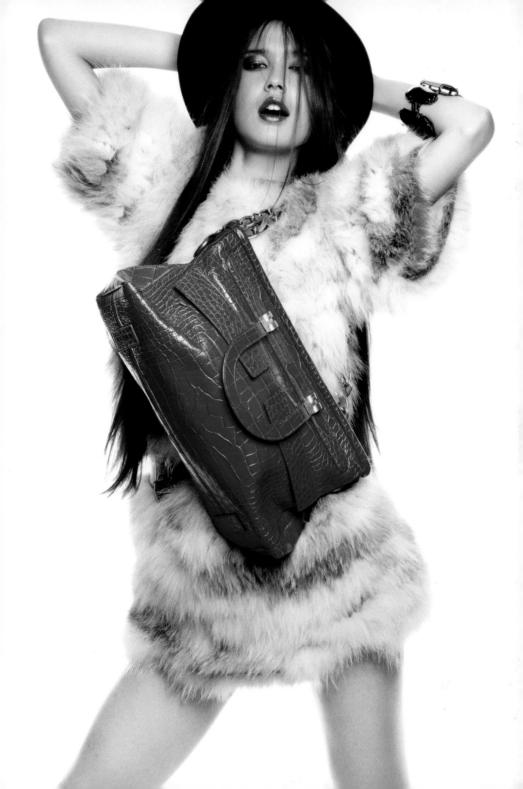

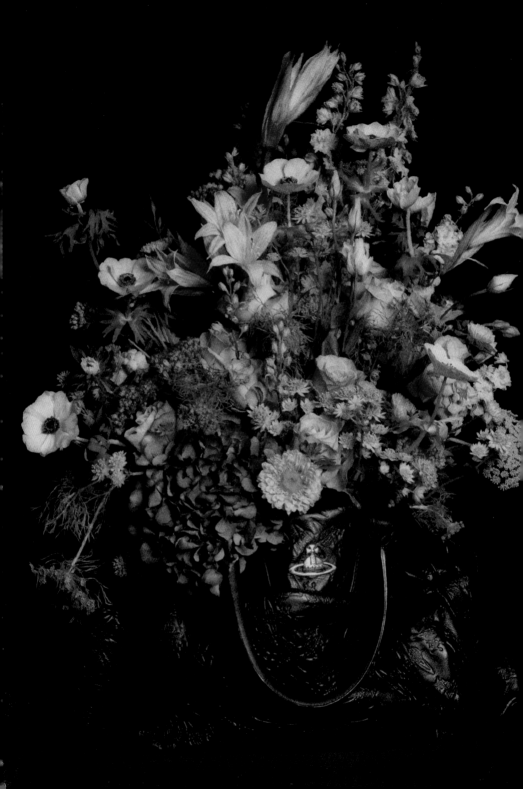

VIVIENNE WESTWOOD

Once considered an outsider, Vivienne
Westwood is now an entrenched part
of the fashion establishment. Her bags
are irreverent interpretations of classic
designs, and are imbued with the punk
spirit for which she is famous.

OPPOSITE Embossed Pier bag, A/W 08/09.

Founded in 1981
www.viviennewestwood.com

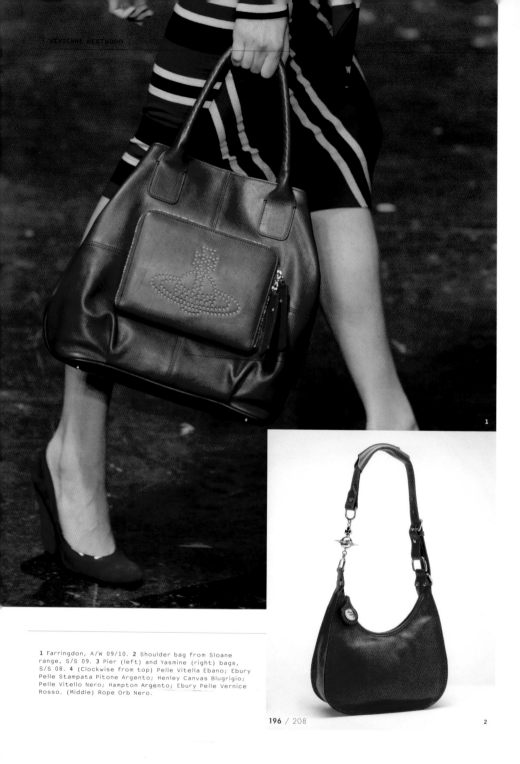

1

1 Farringdon, A/W 09/10. **2** Shoulder bag from Sloane range, S/S 09. **3** Pier (left) and Yasmine (right) bags, S/S 08. **4** (Clockwise from top) Pelle Vitella Ebano; Ebury Pelle Stampata Pitone Argento; Henley Canvas Blugrigio; Pelle Vitello Nero; Hampton Argento; Ebury Pelle Vernice Rosso. (Middle) Rope Orb Nero.

2

CONTROVERSIAL AND CONFRONTATIONAL, WESTWOOD'S DESIGNS MARKED HER AS A FASHION OUTSIDER AND REBEL FROM THE BEGINNING OF HER CAREER.

3

4

Vivienne Westwood is the Grand Dame of British fashion. A living legend, her influence on fashion and culture in the UK cannot be overstated. In her career, which spans over 30 years, she has been an innovator, a rebel and a provocateur, someone with an utterly fearless approach to fashion. Instead of conforming to seasonal trends, she prefers to move forward with her own unique vision, which in turn usually creates its own trends. She is one of the UK's greatest exports and one of the few contemporary designers that have real impact.

Vivienne Westwood first came to the world's attention in the mid-1970s thanks to her shop Sex, located on the Kings Road in London. It's here that she played a major role – along with ex-husband Malcolm McLaren – in the creation of the punk movement. While McLaren managed seminal punk band The Sex Pistols, Westwood designed the semi-bondage clothes that the band wore. It's these clothes that quickly became the uniform of the punk scene. Controversial and confrontational, Westwood's designs marked her as a fashion outsider and rebel from the beginning of her career.

She soon made the transition from rebel to revered. Westwood debuted her Pirate collection in Paris in 1981, making her the first British designer to show in Paris since Mary Quant in the 1960s. Completely self-taught, she constantly pushes the parameters of fashion design. Without the structure of formal training, she has no boundaries or fear when it comes to what can and cannot be accomplished technically in her designs. Working directly on the body and referencing different styles of historical dress, she creates silhouettes that are modern, exciting and innovative.

Although now a firm component of the fashion establishment, Westwood still has a punk attitude. She uses her brand, and specifically her art and design, to highlight some of the world's bigger issues, such as human rights abuses. She may design clothes, but she also wants to stimulate consciousness in her customers.

From humble beginnings in a Kings Road store, Vivienne Westwood is now a global brand that encompasses four clothing lines, five perfumes and over fourteen different product and accessory lines. Vivienne Westwood Bags was launched in 1992, the same year she launched her women's demi-couture 'Gold' line and the 'Red label' diffusion line. Key characteristics of the bags include the use of tartan, a fabric Westwood consistently revisits (she even has her own house tartan), to clever cutting techniques and the use of the metal gold 'orb' logo as a hardware detail or snaffle lock.

The Ebury is perhaps the most widely recognized bag from Westwood's signature bag range, which focuses on luxury designs. An irreverent range of classic styles inspired by the 1950s' Kelly bags, the Ebury bag is a bowling bag shape with structured handles and a large characteristic orb logo detail that comes in fake snake leather or glossy ostrich patent, in a choice of three colourways.

By contrast, the Berkeley bag focuses on pattern, and is an eye-catching range inspired by prints featured in the 'Gold Label' evening gowns. The 'Hampton' is a newly introduced luxury range featuring a gold twist lock Girello fastening.

Bags are more casual in the main collection. The 'Hoxton' is a popular range of sporty nylon shapes – from shoppers and bowling bags to hobo styles – that feature a rope orb print double-runner zip detailing. Also from the main range is the Bettina, a sack-bag shape with knotted handles and metal fittings. The key feature is the detachable orb-embroidered teddybear key ring, which adds a cute touch.

The 'Marina' is a new range of shoppers for Spring/ Summer 09. With a printed check available in four colourways and four different styles of shoppers, all bags feature a leather strap that allows the shoppers to be rolled up so they can be carried easily in another bag.

Vivienne Westwood is one of the last independent brands in the fashion world. Selling in more than 50 countries, she is as relevant now as she was when she started out. Ingrained in British fashion and culture, she continues to innovate as well as to inspire new generations of designers through her bold creations and rebellious spirit.

OPPOSITE The Berkeley bag, A/W 08/09.

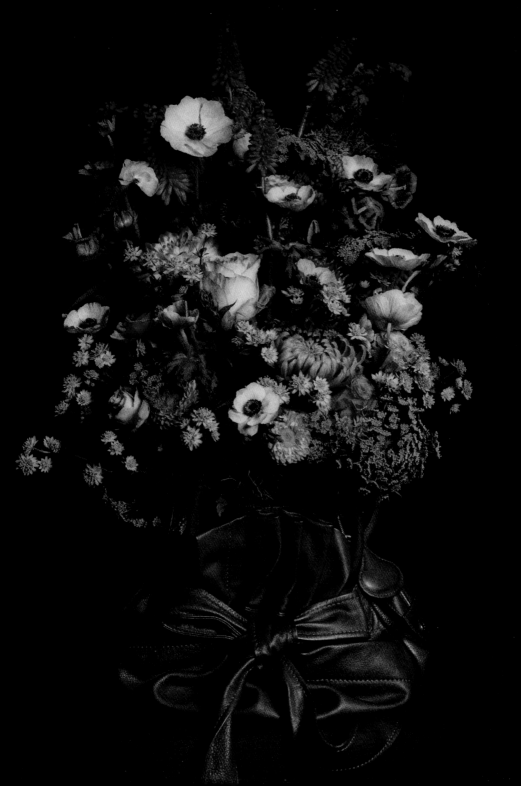

ZAGLIANI

Founded 70 years ago as a company that specialized
in creating luxury bags out of exotic skins,
Zagliani does not follow trends but aims to create
classic, colourful and timeless bags that will be
treasured forever.

OPPOSITE (left) Star clutch in silver spray python,
S/S 09; (right) The Bag 62 in emerald metallic python,
A/W 08/09.

Founded in 1947
www.zagliani.it

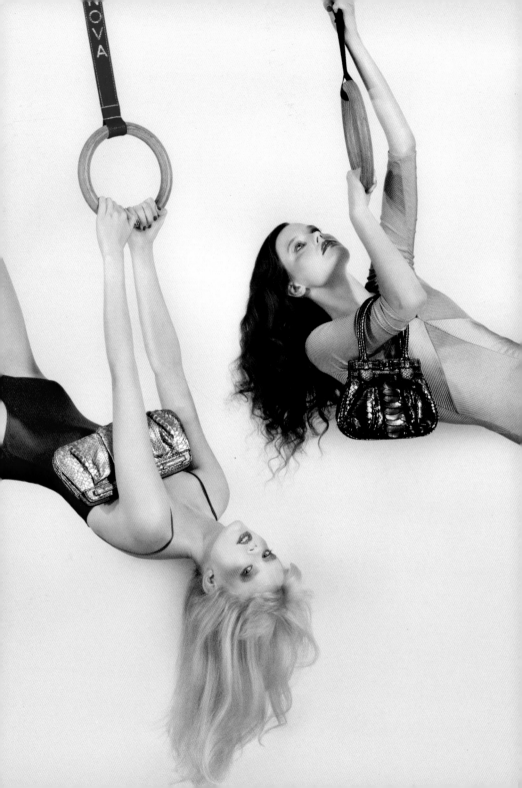

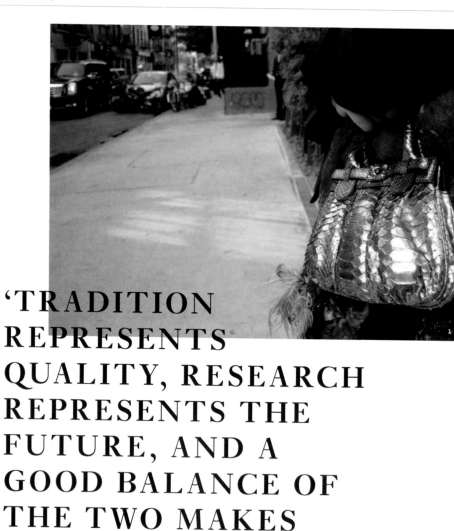

'TRADITION REPRESENTS QUALITY, RESEARCH REPRESENTS THE FUTURE, AND A GOOD BALANCE OF THE TWO MAKES THE PERFECT BAG'

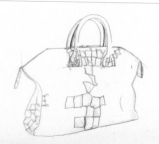

1 The Bag 62 in gold metallic python, S/S 08. 2 Sketch of the Tomodachi crocodile bag, S/S 07. 3 Yume bag in natural python, A/W 07/08. 4 Pleat bag in ice-grey python, A/W 07/08. 5 Pleat bag in marron glace lizard, A/W 08/09. 6 Puffy bag 04 in 18ct gold python, A/W 08/09.

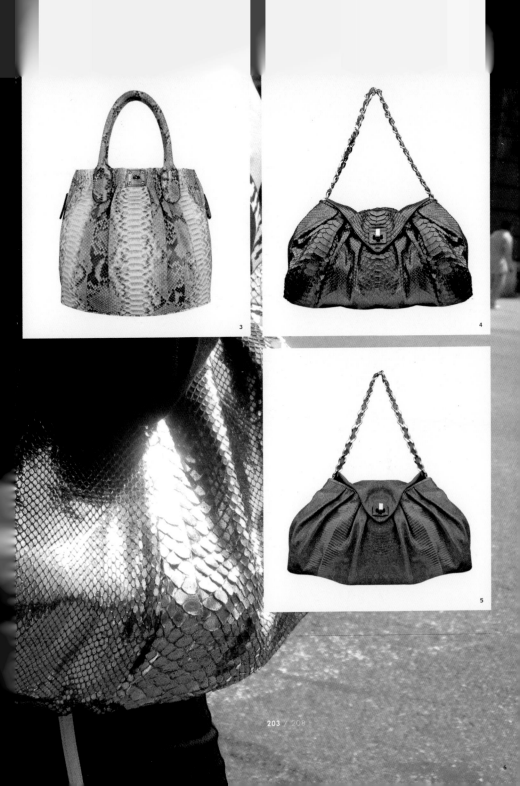

3

4

5

6

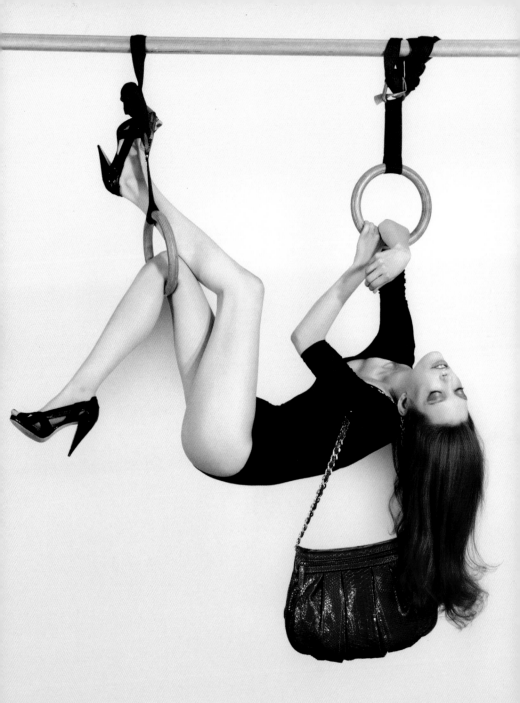

Milan-based Zagliani, established in the 1940s by its namesake Bruna Zagliani, was relaunched in 2006 with the help of creative talent Mauro Orietti-Carella. By linking the heritage of Zagliani with future-oriented research, Orietti-Carella successfully created the perfect marriage between tradition and technology.

Whether by chance, by accident or

'because it was written in my stars',

Orietti-Carella's entry into the world of handbag design was not as clearly defined as some.

'Initially, I wasn't really attracted to the world of handbags. To be honest I thought it was too boring.'

However, after acting as a consultant for the brand, Orietti-Carella become enchanted by Zagliani's heritage and ended up buying the company when it ran into financial difficulties.

Having spent his formative years living in the Far East, Orietti-Carella has learnt the importance of viewing the world from different perspectives. This philosophy inspired him to bring his previous medical expertise as a dermatologist to his career in fashion, which resulted in a new design phase for the Zagliani brand.

Recognizing the similarities in both human- and crocodile skin, notably the need to keep both soft and hydrated, Orietti-Carella began injecting exotic crocodile skins with silicone and resins. The result was remarkable – materials become lighter, stronger and softer to the touch.

'My formula puts an end to traditional stiff crocodile bags and creates soft, extremely strong contemporary accessories',

explains Orietti-Carella.

Technology aside, the design process remains extremely important to Orietti-Carella. It starts with what he considers the most important step, selecting a colour palette:

'It is a long process, perhaps the longest one in creating a new collection.'

Citing the artist Rothko as one of his greatest influences, Orietti-Carella is inspired by his great sensibility and love of creating new shades and combinations:

'Colour is the main element of my work, this is so important to me because I use colours to communicate a concept, to design a story.'

Part of the process involves painting the skins (which are ethically sourced) until the right shades are achieved.

When the colours have been selected, prototypes are then constructed using paper.

'I don't really design bags at the beginning, instead I create a prototype in paper so I am able to visualize proportion, sizes and shape.'

Once the prototypes are established, Orietti-Carella sets about defining the finer details of the design.

'I design the collection only when I have been able to find the perfect proportions in at least two new prototypes out of the four or five styles I have created. I tend to break what I consider the "classic proportions" in order to give my collections a new perspective.'

Despite all of these innovations, Orietti-Carella and Zagliani work hard to ensure that they do not lose sight of the market.

'When making luxury bags it is not enough to buy expensive skins and add a logo. The market is more mature, the customer understands good quality and is certainly more individually minded. They want to feel unique',

explains Orietti-Carella. This is not always an easy task to achieve, but being unique is a reality Zagliani already has written in its DNA.

Traditionally, Zagliani is known for manufacturing handbags in exotic skins and, while this is still very much the ethos of the brand, Orietta-Carella sees himself as the link between the past and future. However, rather than plunder the archives and re-imagine, he is careful to continue the tradition of craftsmanship by highlighting strong and unique details that say quality and individuality. In the designer's own words:

'you don't buy a Zagliani bag for its logo. You buy it because you, as an individual, can recognize its beauty. After all, I am just trying to make beautiful bags.'

OPPOSITE Puffy with chain handle in ruby python, A/W 08/09.

The authors and publisher would like to thank the following institutions and individuals for providing photographic images for use in this book. In all cases every effort has been made to credit the copyright holders, but should there be any omissions or errors the publisher would be pleased to insert the appropriate acknowledgment in any subsequent edition of this book.

ANYA HINDMARCH
p12&17 Photography by John-Paul Pietrus · Retouching and digital artwork by Nick Nedeljkovic at Happy Finish
p14&4 and p15&7 Photography by Steven Emberton
All other images courtesy of Anya Hindmarch

BOTKIER
p19 Photography by John-Paul Pietrus · Styling by Natalie Wansbrough-Jones · Hair by Kenichi at Caren · Make-up by Adam de Cruz at Balcony Jump · Model: Dustin at FM · Retouching and digital artwork by Nick Nedeljkovic at Happy Finish
All other images by Monica Botkier © Botkier Inc

BULGA
p24 Photography by John-Paul Pietrus · Styling by Niki Brodie · Hair by Asashi at Caren · Make-up by Adam de Cruz at Balcony Jump · Models: Alina and Anzhela at Storm, Govan at Premier, Wanessa at Select · Retouching and digital artwork by Nick Nedeljkovic at Happy Finish · p31 She wears clothes by Jitrois; girls wear gold dress (worn under fur gilet, stylist's own), vintage Thierry Mugler, Decades at Dover Street Market; gunmetal metallic dress and silk nude dress with Swarovski crystal detail, both by Bodyamr
All other images courtesy of Bulga

BURBERRY
p31&34 Photography by John-Paul Pietrus · Styling by Georgia Ashdown www.georgiaashdown.com · Hair by Joel Goncalves at Naked Artists for John Frieda Salons · Make-up by Liz Martins at Naked Artists · Manicure by Kim Treacy · Models: Betty at Models 1 and Rainer at Select · Retouching and digital artwork by Nick Nedeljkovic at Happy Finish · p31 She wears Body Armour body suit, Sophie Huline sequin hood, Roberto Cavalli ring, Maria Francesca Pepe necklace (worn as belt); he wears Richard James briefs · p34 She wears Tina Kalivas dress, Chatila earrings and ring; he wears Acne trousers, Dior sunglasses
All other images courtesy of Burberry

CHANEL
p36&42-43 Photography by John-Paul Pietrus · Styling by Joan Campbell www.joancampbell.co.uk · Hair by Asashi at Caren · Make-up by Liz Martins at Naked Artists · Manicure by Lucie Pickavance at Caren · Model: Kine Diouf at Independent · Retouching and digital artwork by Nick Nedeljkovic at Happy Finish
p38&39 #1,#3 ©CHANEL; #2 ©CHANEL, sketch — Karl Lagerfeld · p41 #1,#3 ©CHANEL; #2 ©CHANEL, photograph — Karl Lagerfeld

CHARLOTT VASBERG
p45&49: Photography by John-Paul Pietrus · Styling by Tim Lim · Hair by Chen Tao · Make-up by Wang Qian · Models: Sun Fei Fei at Elite, Zhang Xu Chao, Du Shi Bao, Wang Jiang · Photographic assistance by Guo Liang · Styling assistance by Tang Shuang · Production by Mia Chen and Jian Cui · p45 Vintage dresses by Herve Leger · p49 She wears vintage dress by Herve Leger; he wears turtleneck and suit by Giorgio Armani
All other images courtesy of Charlott Vasberg/Inger Ltd · Photography by Thomas Odulate · Styling by Amber Brierley

CHLOÉ
p50&54: Photography by John-Paul Pietrus · Styling by Alice Giannini www.alicegiannini.com · Hair by Asashi at Caren · Make-up by Adam de Cruz at Balcony Jump · Manicure by Sarka · Model: Rosie Snowden at Select · Retouching and digital artwork by Nick Nedeljkovic at Happy Finish · p50 (top) silver fox fur stole by Hockley, nude bodysuit by Prada, Swarovski crystal costume cuff and necklace both from a selection at Alfie's Antiques; (bottom) pink silk puff jacket by Roksanda Ilincic, nude bodysuit by Prada, silver and crystal cuff from Alfie's Antiques · p54 (top) dark green fur coat by Gerard Darel, nude bodysuit by Prada; (bottom) nude bodysuit by Prada
p53 #1 Photography by Dan Leca; #2,#3 Photography by Wilfred Gremillet; #4,#5 Courtesy of Chloé

CORTO MOLTEDO
p57&61 Photography by John-Paul Pietrus · Styling by Joan Campbell www.joancampbell.co.uk · Hair by Joel Gonçalves at Naked Artists · Make-up by Liz Martins at Naked Artists · Manicure by Lucie Pickavance at Caren · Model: Petr at Select · Retouching and digital artwork by Nick Nedeljkovic at Happy Finish · Hayabusa bike courtesy of Mark Law, Mark Hamey and Beanos Nuts www.beanos-nuts.co.uk · Denim shirt and jeans both by Nudie Jeans Co, glasses by Yves Saint Laurent
All other images courtesy of Corto Moltedo

DOLCE&GABBANA
p62&68: Photography by John-Paul Pietrus · Styling by Oxana Korsun · Hair by Kenichi at Caren · Make-up by Adam de Cruz at Balcony Jump · Manicure by Lucie Pickavance at Caren · Model: Hyoni Kang at Independent · She wears dress by Dolce&Gabbana
All other images courtesy of Dolce&Gabbana

ERVA
p71&75: Photography by John-Paul Pietrus · Styling by Niki Brodie · Hair by Asashi at Caren · Make-up by Adam de Cruz at Balcony Jump · Models: Govan at Premier and Alina at Storm · Retouching and digital artwork by Nick Nedeljkovic at Happy Finish · p71 She wears gold strapless dress, vintage Thierry Mugler, Decades at Dover Street Market. He wears dinner jacket, shirt and bowtie, all by Gieves & Hawkes · p75 She wears tuxedo jacket, by Ann-Sofie Back. He wears dinner jacket and shirt, both by Gieves & Hawkes
All other images courtesy of Erva

HALSTON
p76&82 Photography by John-Paul Pietrus · Hair by Kenichi at Caren · Make-up by Adam de Cruz at Balcony Jump · Model: Iekeliene at Select · Retouching and digital artwork by Nick Nedeljkovic at Happy Finish
p79 #1,#2, Don Ashby; #3 courtesy of Halston
p80&81 All images courtesy of Halston · Photography by Ted Morrison

HERMÈS
p85&88: Photography by John-Paul Pietrus · Retouching and digital artwork by Nick Nedeljkovic at Happy Finish
All other images courtesy of Hermès (GB) Ltd

ISAAC REINA
p90&97 Photography by John-Paul Pietrus · Manicure by Lucie Pickavance at Caren · Hand and Foot Model: Sarah Lloyd at Hired Hands · Retouching and digital artwork by Nick Nedeljkovic at Happy Finish
p93 Shop image by Alfredo Salazar
All other images courtesy of Isaac Reina · Photography by Carles A. Roig

JAMIN PUECH
p99&103 Photography by John-Paul Pietrus · Manicure by Sharka · Hand model: Sarah Lloyd at Hired Hands
All other images courtesy of Isabelle Puech and Benoît Jamin · Photography by Wilfred Gremillet

JAS M.B.
p104&109 Photography by John-Paul Pietrus · Styling by Joan Campbell www.joancampbell.co.uk · Hair by Joel Gonçalves at Naked Artists · Make-up by Liz Martins at Naked Artists · Manicure by Lucie Pickavance at Caren · Model: Tamara Moss at IMG
All other images courtesy of Jas M.B.

JÉRÔME DREYFUSS
p111&114 Photography by John-Paul Pietrus · Styling by Georgia Ashdown www.georgiaashdown.com · Hair by Kenichi at Caren · Make-up by Adam de Cruz at Balcony Jump · Manicure by Lucie Pickavance at Caren · Model: Rahma at IMG · Retouching and digital artwork by Nick Nedeljkovic at Happy Finish · p111 She wears Just Cavalli coat, Alexis Bittar rings · p114 She wears Metallicus body stocking, Roberto Cavalli ring, Iceburg leather gloves
All other images courtesy of Jérôme Dreyfuss

KAVIAR GAUCHE
p116&121 Photography by John-Paul Pietrus · Styling by Joan Campbell www.joancampbell.co.uk · Hair by Joel Gonçalves at Naked Artists · Make-up by Liz Martins at Naked Artists · Manicure by Lucie Pickavance at Caren · Model: Isa at Select
All other images courtesy of Alexandra Fischer Roehler and Johanna Kühl

LARA BOHINC
p123&126 Photography by John-Paul Pietrus · Hair by Ben Mohopi · Make-up by Kim Kiefer · Manicure by Sarka · Model: Karolina Mikolajczyk at Next · Retouching and digital artwork by Nick Nedeljkovic at Happy Finish
All other images courtesy of Lara Bohinc; photography by Jernej Prelac www.jernejprelac.com

LIBERTY OF LONDON
p128&132 Photography by John-Paul Pietrus · Styling by Georgia Ashdown www.georgiaashdown.com · Hair by Kenichi at Caren · Make-up by Adam de Cruz at Balcony Jump · Manicure by Lucie Pickavance at Caren · Model: Rahma at IMG · Retouching and digital artwork by Nick Nedeljkovic at Happy Finish · She wears Camilla Staerk lace and silk dress with train, Alexis Bittar earrings and rings, fake tights, stylist's own shoes
All other images courtesy of Liberty of London

LOEWE
p135&140 Photography by John-Paul Pietrus · Styling by Oxana Korsun · Hair by Kenichi at Caren · Make-up by Adam de Cruz at Balcony Jump · Manicure by Lucie Pickavance at Caren · Model: Lekeliene Stange at Select · Retouching and digital artwork by Nick Nedeljkovic at Happy Finish · p135 She wears vintage Agnes B blouse, trousers by Cacharel, vintage belt and scarf · p140 She wears shirt by COS, poloneck by Uniqlo, trousers by Loewe
All other images courtesy of Loewe

MARC JACOBS
p142&147 Photography by John-Paul Pietrus · Hair by Ben Mohopi · Make-up by Angela Davis Deacon at Naked Artists · Manicure by Sarka · Model: Karolina Mikolajczyk at Next · Retouching and digital artwork by Nick Nedeljkovic at Happy Finish
All other images courtesy of Marc Jacobs

MOSCHINO
p149&152 Photography by John-Paul Pietrus · Styling by Georgia Ashdown www.georgiaashdown.com · Hair by Kenichi at Caren · Make-up by Adam de Cruz at Balcony Jump · Manicure by Lucie Pickavance at Caren · Model: Rahma at IMG · p149 She wears Christian Dior fishnet tights, Charlotte Dellal ankle boots · p152 She wears Wolford neon orange tights, Pierre Hardy patent heels p150&151 #1,#2,#3 courtesy of Moschino, photography by Riccardo Vimercati; #4,#5 courtesy of Moschino, photography by Matteo Oriani and Raffaele Origone

PAURIC SWEENEY
p154&159 Photography by John-Paul Pietrus · Styling by Alice Giannini www.alicegiannini.com · Hair by Asashi at Caren · Make-up by Adam de Cruz at Balcony Jump · Manicure by Sarka · Model: Victoria S at Models 1 · Retouching and digital artwork by Nick Nedeljkovic at Happy Finish · p154 She wears camel coat and trousers by Kisa · p159 She wears black kimono-style dress by Hermés
All other images courtesy of Pauric Sweeney

3.1 PHILLIP LIM
p161&166 Photography by John-Paul Pietrus · Styling by Tim Lim · Hair by Chen Tao · Make-up by Wang Qian · Model: Du Juan at Ink Pak · Photographic assistance by Guo Liang · Styling assistance by Tang Shuang · Production by Mia Chen and Jian Cui · Retouching and digital artwork by Nick Nedeljkovic at Happy Finish · p161 She wears dress by Maison Martin Margiela; bodysuit by Wolford · p166 She wears sequin jacket by CHANEL; bodysuit by Wolford; boots by Yves Saint Laurent
p162 Photography by Henry Han · p165 Photography by Kelly Bruggema · p163 Photography by Carlotta Manaigo
All other images courtesy of Phillip Lim

PIERRE HARDY
p168&173 photography by John-Paul Pietrus · Hair by Kenichi at Caren · Make-up by Adam de Cruz at Balcony Jump · Model: Edward Barber at FM · Retouching and digital artwork by Nick Nedeljkovic at Happy Finish
All other images courtesy of Pierre Hardy

PORTS 1961
p175&178 Photography by John-Paul Pietrus
All other images courtesy of Ports 1961

ROCIO
p180&186 Photography by John-Paul Pietrus · Styling by Joan Campbell www.joancampbell.co.uk · Hair by Asashi at Caren · Make-up by Liz Martins at Naked Artists · Manicure by Lucie Pickavance at Caren · Model: Kine Diouf at Independent · Retouching and digital artwork by Nick Nedeljkovic at Happy Finish · Deer talent supplied by David Mills +44(0) 1342 834 658 · p180 She wears printed silk dress from Rellik · p186 She wears organza printed dress by Ossie Clark, sandals from Rellik
All other images courtesy of Hamish Menzies, Thessa Nepomuceno and Rocio Olbes
Rocio is a registered trademark of Rocio Ltd. © 2009 Rocio Ltd.UK

VERSACE
p189&193 Photography by John-Paul Pietrus · Styling by Georgia Ashdown www.georgiaashdown.com · Hair by Joel Goncalves at Naked Artists for John Frieda Salons · Make-up by Liz Martins at Naked Artists · Manicure by Kim Treacy · Model: Mirhe at IMG · Retouching and digital artwork by Nick Nedeljkovic at Happy Finish · p189 She wears Roberto Cavalli fur, Liza Bruce swimsuit, Chatilla ring and bracelet, Burberry cuff, Chatilla necklace · p193 She wears Hans Madsen fur dress, Nogoy belt from Liberty, Burberry cluster bracelet, Roberto Cavalli gold necklace, Lock & Co felt hat
All other images courtesy of Versace

VIVIENNE WESTWOOD
p194&199 Photography by John-Paul Pietrus · Floral arrangements created by Phllo Flowers www.phlloflowers.com · Retouching and digital artwork by Nick Nedeljkovic at Happy Finish
All other images courtesy of Vivienne Westwood Ltd

ZAGLIANI
p201&204 Photography by John-Paul Pietrus · Styling by Joan Campbell www.joancampbell.co.uk · Hair by Joel Goncalves at Naked Artists · Make-up by Liz Martins at Naked Artists · Manicure by Lucie Pickavance at Caren · Models: Isa, Kerrie and Ellie at Select · Set designed by Andrea Cellerino · Retouching and digital artwork by Nick Nedeljkovic at Happy Finish · Bodies by Repetto, shoes by Amanda Wakeley
Street Photography by Mauro Orietti-Carella
All other images courtesy of Zagliani

p208 Image provided by CHANEL, ©Assouline

Author's dedications:
Sue Huey would like to dedicate this book to her daughter, Iris Mae Fraser.
Susie Draffan dedicates this book to her gran.

The publisher would like to offer sincere thanks to all of the designers who have contributed to this book, and to all of their personnel who have assisted in supplying information and images.

Sue Huey and Susie Draffan would like to thank Gaynor Sermon, Helen Evans, Jay Hess, Simone Pasztorek and John-Paul Pietrus, without whose hard work, dedication and perseverance this book would not have been possible. Thanks also to Alison Bishop and Claire Murphy for all their help in organizing the photography shoots.

Sue would also like to specially thank Graeme for all his help and support, and dedicates this book to her daughter, Iris Mae Fraser.

Susie would also like to give special thanks to her mum and dad for always supporting and inspiring her, and to Ellie and Claire for being great sounding boards.

John-Paul Pietrus would like to thank:

Amanda Kelly and Peri Mosig from NAKED ARTISTS who represent make-up artists Liz Martins and Angela Davis Deacon, hair stylist Joel Gonçalves and Nail technician Kim Treacy www.nakedartists.com · Caren Fisk and Gaelle Lecomte from CAREN who represent hair stylists Asashi and Kenichi and nail technician Lucie Pickavance www.caren.co.uk · Candice O'Brien from BALCONY JUMP who represent make-up artist Adam de Cruz www.balconyjump.co.uk · Hair stylists Benjamin Mohapi www.benjaminmohapi.com and Chen Tao · Make-up artists Kim Kiefer www.kimkiefer.co.uk and Wang Qian · Nail technician Sharka

Hannah Sneath, Ben Yuen, Ian Loughran, Sarah Leon, Dounia Benjelloul from SELECT MODEL MANAGEMENT who represent Lekeliene Stange, Wanessa, Rosie Snowden, Kerrie, Ellie, Isa, Rainer and Petr www.selectmodel.com · Debbie Jones and Katy Lyons from MODELS 1 who represent Victoria Sekrier www.models1.co.uk · Nina from FIERCE who represents Elizabeth · Noelle Doukas from STORM MODELS who represents Alina and Anzhela www.stormmodels.com · Stephen Jollife and Ash Mosley from FM MODEL AGENCY who represent Edward Barber and Dustin www.fmmodelagency.com · Khalid El-Awad from IMG MODELS who represents Rahma, Mirhe and Tamara Moss www.imgmodels.com · Jamie Horridge from INDEPENDENT TALENT who represents Kinee Diouf and Hyoni Kang www.independenttalent.com · Christophe Sanchez-Vahle from PREMIER MODEL MANAGEMENT who represents Govan www.premiermodelmanagement.com · Melvin Chua from INK PAK who represents Du Juan · Versae Vanni from NEXT MODELS who represents Karolina www.nextmodels.com · CHINA MODELS who represent Sun Fei Fei, Zhang Xu Chao, Du Shi Bao, Wang Jiang · HIRED HANDS who represent Sarah Lloyd www.hiredhandsmodels.com

Fashion editors: Georgia Ashdown www.georgiaashdown.com · Niki Brodie www.nikibrodie@mac.com · Joan Campbell www.joancampbell.co.uk · Alice Gianinni www.alicegiannini.com · Natalie Wansbrough-Jones · Oxana Korsun · Tim Lim

Nick Nedeljkovic from Happy Finish for retouching and digital artwork www.happyfinish.net and thanks also to Richard Tisdall

Special thanks to Provision, for providing digital equipment and technicians www.provisionphotographic.com

Special thanks to Sola Studios www.solalights.com

Special thanks to Mark Law and Mark Hamey from Beanos Nuts for providing the Hayabusa in the Corto Moltedo chapter www.beanos-nuts.co.uk

Interns: Roel van Koppenhagen, Megan Smith and Linda McLaughlin

Special thanks: Emanuele Titomanlio, Duro Olowu, Roksanda Ilincic, Zoe Olive, Mia Chen, Jian Cui, Eka Yu, Tang Shuang, Guo Liang, AJ Numan and Sam Jackson

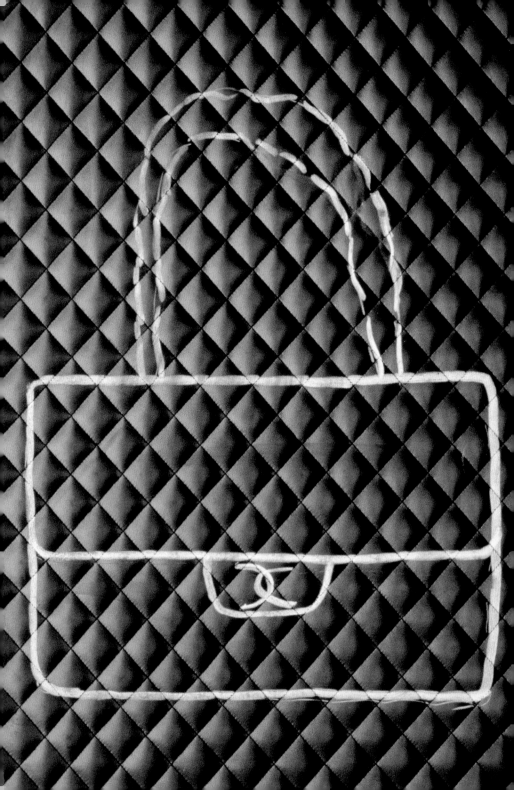